What Pharmacists Are Saying

"If you are a student, pharmacist, or other health professional who's feeling stuck, overwhelmed, or wanting to meaningfully reimagine what's next, this is the book for you. Unscripted On Purpose *is a real, vulnerable window into one pharmacist's faith-filled journey to living her fullest purpose-driven life. This book will challenge, inspire, and empower you with practical tips/tools, and tug at the places of your heart that need to be reawakened, or even discovered for the first time, moving you to take intentional next steps in becoming all you were made to be, personally and professionally."*

—**Rachel Firebaugh,** PharmD, Faculty at University of Washington, USA

"Katrina takes you on her professional and personal journey as a pharmacist to help you discover how you are called to more, giving you practical steps along the way to discover your purpose, passion, and calling. Pharmacists in varying stages of their careers will resonate with the stories and principles in the book."

—**Justin Cole,** PharmD, USA

"Valuable to health professionals, especially pharmacists, at all stages of their life and career journeys. This is a very holistic approach, which includes faith-based values, and creates a unique approach to reflection and evaluation of our experiences and pathways."

—**Kay Dunkley,** Pharmacist, CEO - Pharmacist Support Services, Australia

"A toolkit to help pharmacists break free, out of the box, and create their own career path that is meaningful to them and aligned with their values. An empowering permission slip to dream BIG and beyond what society and faculties expect of pharmacists."

—**Julie Doan,** PharmD, Certified Coach, Canada

"This book genuinely moved me. It resonated deeply with the quiet reflections many pharmacists share but rarely articulate: the tension between purpose and productivity, care and compliance. Reading it felt like holding up a mirror to my own journey. It equipped me with the language and courage to reframe my "Call to More." Most importantly, it delivers on its promise. It doesn't just remind pharmacists why our work matters; it helps us reconnect with how it matters through compassion, curiosity, and the continual reimagining of our role in a changing healthcare landscape."

—**Ayomide Ogundipe,** Pharmaceutical Society of Australia Early-Career Pharmacist Board Director, Australia

A Journey and Purpose-Driven Guide for Pharmacists Who Feel Called to More

Unscripted ON PURPOSE

Katrina Azer

Unscripted On Purpose

Published by Unscripted by Kat

ISBN (hardback): 978-1-0671195-2-2
ISBN (paperback): 978-1-0671195-9-1

Cover design by Alan Hebel

Dedicated to
the unsung hero in the white coat
the pharmacist who feels called to more.

PREFACE

Unscripted

adj.

To be unwritten and unbound—no longer confined to the scripts handed down by tradition or society. A way of living that dares to replace certainty with curiosity, safety with courage, and expectation with truth. To be Unscripted is to walk a path of purpose that unfolds step by step, where faith steadies the unknown and meaning is discovered, not prescribed.

Pharmacist

n.

An entrusted steward of medications who purposefully and courageously resists systems that overuse them, reclaiming medicines as tools for healing, never instruments of harm. A clinician trained in the quality use of medicines, yet called to compassion and human connection. A professional whose title opens the door to a deeper vocation—one grounded in hope, practiced in patient service, and lived out in a life of meaning and purpose that extends far beyond medicines.

Dear Pharmacist Who Feels Called to More,

I thought I had reached the height of success, and that it would make me happy. The credentials, the awards… Yes, I got them; yet the ache was soul-deep. What unsettled me most was not knowing why. My colleagues envied me, even called me "ungrateful," because after years of rejection and clawing my way forward, I had finally "made it." Yet, in the quiet of my own heart, I still asked, *Is this it?*

Hi, I'm Katrina. Though my degree calls me a pharmacist, my heart has always been searching for something deeper—a life where work is not just survival but an expression of meaning and purpose. And if you've ever felt this restless pursuit, this book is for you.

In 2020, I nearly collapsed on the pharmacy floor because my body couldn't take it any longer. Like many of you, balancing work and life, I had used all my sick days and was too afraid to request a day off. For thirteen years, I bore the burden of a broken system until it broke me too. Eventually, I asked myself, "Is this worth my health?" and I walked away.

Only later did I realize that burnout is a symptom of misalignment—when values and ambitions are chained to a system that grants us no agency and measures worth by script volumes rather than health outcomes. That was the moment I knew I had to own my fate. I began to ask bigger questions: *Why am I here on earth? What if my purpose is more than this title?*

Countless pharmacists have asked me, "How did you get here? How did you get so lucky?" My reply is simple: I refused to accept the complacency of the narrative society defines for us. I didn't get "lucky." I listened to my intuition, refused to follow the script handed down to me, and chose the Unscripted path to freedom, fulfillment, and purpose. Now, I want to share the path that brought me here with you. This isn't a book about my life; it's a book that borrows my life to hand yours back to you. I wrote it not because I have all the answers, but because I walked through the fire and found my way back to a more purposeful career and life.

I wrote this book for pharmacists who, like I once was, are searching for their soul purpose. For those who yearn for more, chasing credentials, validation, or money, yet finding that none of it fills the hollow inside. For those seeking a truer path to fulfillment. For the burned-out and the weary who long for healing. And for those who have reached the apex and still feel "not enough," or who have done all the "right" things in their career and still whisper, *Is this it?*

I extend my deepest gratitude to those who carried me here, from you, the reader, who invested in this book, to the beta readers, editor, cover designer, and every person who touched this journey. Yes, even those who rejected me: your "no" redirected me to my purpose. For all of it, thank you!

Pharmacist: This is your permission to find your Call to More, and your why.

Because…

"He who has a 'why' to live can bear almost any 'how.'"

— Friedrich Nietzsche

May these pages reignite the calling inside you.

With love and purpose,

Katrina

CONTENTS

INTRODUCTION

How This Unscripted Guide Will Walk With You

If you picked up this book because the script handed to you has withered away, then you're in the right place. And yes, there is another script waiting to be written.

As you dive through the pages of this book, I want you to know and believe this:

"You were created on purpose, for a purpose."

I know the inner critic too well. It seizes on your lowest moments—bad days at work, career fails, layoffs, colleagues who betray, words that cut at your worth and character, whispering, *You don't matter.* That is a lie. You do matter. And your existence is no coincidence. You are here on purpose and for a purpose. The truth that freed me was simple but profound: My job and my social standing do not determine my worth. My role on Earth is not to fit the mold society designed for me. It is to step into the purpose I was created for—to reach the highest potential God has destined me for in the service of others, that which is aligned with His calling. And that, friends, only happens when you live life *Unscripted, On Purpose*—a journey this book will invite you into with honesty, courage, and grace.

A Word on Faith

I know pharmacists from many faiths and worldviews will read this book. But I will be honest with you: This is a Christian faith-based, purpose-driven book. I would not be here, and these words would not exist, without God's strength, "For in Him we live and move and have our being" (Acts 17:28 NIV). Before this book came to be, it was only blank pages, a whispered prayer at a kitchen table: *God, if there's more, then show me the next right step.* Despite every challenge I encountered while writing this, He gave me the strength to keep going. I pray it might help you find your way back to clarity, purpose, and meaning beyond the boundaries of your career. (If you want to find out more about my faith, see the appendix.)

How to Use This Book

This is not a book you read, but one you interact with.
Inside, you'll find:

- **Pro-Tips** → margin callouts with practical advice, resources, and encouragement.
- **Reflections** → mid-chapter reflection prompts to help you pause and put the chapter into your own words.
- **Unscript Yourself Echoes** → mid- and end-of-chapter reflections, inner nudges, bold truths, and reframes woven through Chapters 1–12, to help you merge identity and purpose and actually stop, listen, and write your own next step.
- **Faith Echoes** → optional end-of-chapter moments woven through Chapters 1–12, where I process things through my relationship with God. If that's not your language, you're still welcome here. Let it speak to you or skip it; either way, this journey is yours too.
- **Unscript Yourself Toolkits** → practical end-of-chapter action guides at the end of Chapters 1–12, with journaling prompts that help with career, clarity, reinvention, and finding your Call to More.
- **Unscripted Permission Slips and Affirmations** → short, compassionate declarations that release guilt, restore agency and boundaries, and re-anchor your identity as a human and a healer.

- **Unscripted Tips** → practical resources that supported me along this journey.

From Chapter 13 onward, including the Letters section, you'll notice that the above elements are intentionally absent because the pace slows so you can sit with the invitation rather than rush to fix yourself.

Remember:

- Echoes stir the heart.
- Toolkits shift the steps.
- Faith Echoes keep you rooted.

This book is divided into five parts, each containing chapters that mirror the phases of my Unscripted career. The final part, Part Six, draws the strands together to help you find your Call to More. Lastly comes the Epilogue Series—a section that is not where the story ends, but where the walk begins. It consists of short letters that are trail markers. Return to them when you meet resistance, and revisit them when you need courage. They are lessons I'm still living now.

You can skip the echoes and toolkits if you wish, but since this is a purpose-driven guide, I encourage you to linger with them. They will help consolidate the message, offer clarity, and provide practical steps as you begin to get *Unscripted On Purpose*.

I hope that, by following the chronology of my career path, you see that the Call to More is not answered by following a script, but by merging with life itself—by leaning on intuition, purpose, and meaning at every step. I did not write this book to hand you answers, but to walk beside you as you discover your own.

A Final Word of Permission

You are not just a pharmacist. You are meant for more. It is okay for you to seek it and claim it. This book will give you permission to pursue your calling and to remember that you are more than the role or title you've been handed.

My prayer is that by the end of this book, you will have a renewed sense of identity beyond the title, that you will dare to live life *Unscripted On Purpose*, and that you will find your Call to More—fulfillment, meaning, and purpose in your career and life.

Let's begin the journey.

Katrina

PART I

The Origin

"Rejection is redirection."

—BRYANT MCGILL

CHAPTER 1

You Are Meant for More Than the Script

When we give up on our dreams,
we die while still alive.

—Robin Sharma

I felt devastated. Four years of my life seemed to have culminated in nothing but despair. Exams were done and dusted, the ink barely dry on the answer sheets, and yet here I was, the only one without an internship (preregistration) position secured.

It was five years earlier, on an uneventful evening, when my father exclaimed, "Just do pharmacy." I think he trusted I knew what I was doing with my life. The truth is, I didn't! I muffled an "okay" with complete resolve for several reasons you may relate to. First, pharmacy was a safe option. Second, I was raised with the mindset of "thou shalt obey thy parents." However, as I progressed in my career, I learned that my obedience was, in fact, a hindrance, and the good-girl veneer cracked. I became more of a rebel against the status quo, not out of principle, but out of an exhaustion so deep that I stopped caring what would happen to me if I spoke up. Finally, and most importantly, I had experience working in a community pharmacy over the summer holidays, and I loved the patient connection.

Even when I worked there as a shop assistant, some patients came back asking for me, assuming I was the pharmacist. That trust stirred something in me. There's something sacred at play when a patient steps into a pharmacy, hands you their script and symptoms, and shares their story—all without you asking. Moreover, it didn't "look" like an onerous job. *Squiggling on those prescriptions had always looked so easy.*

All right, I'll admit it . . . because I know you will connect with this on a soul-deep level. I buried some dreams in the name of earning a degree. After working those summers in retail pharmacy, what I wanted to be was a makeup artist. I loved makeup artistry and still do: the shimmering eyeshadow palettes, the lipsticks to suit any mood, and the way a brush could transform not only a face but a person's confidence. All that glamorous promise lit something within me. Though just picturing the look on my father's face if I'd said I wanted to be a makeup artist was enough to shut that dream down before it ever got airtime.

Just as one forbidden dream reminds me of the others I buried next to it, my mind wanders further back. What I wanted more than blending contour lines was to be a Hollywood actress. I've had that dream since childhood. I used to snag all the lead roles in school productions—not because I was the loudest (though, fair point), but because I was actually good. Drama teachers told me I was a natural and should consider acting as a career…but alas! Maybe you've got your own "but alas" too—the talent that was whispered over you by teachers or friends, only to be smothered by culture, duty, or fear.

Now, if telling my father I wanted to be a makeup artist caused a minor earthquake, then telling him I wanted to be an actress? Well, that would've been nuclear! All it would take is one mental image of his daughter kissing a random dude on screen, and *boom!* Every tradition, every cultural line drawn in concrete, would've vanished. He would have disowned me.

I'm sure you have that creative spark in you, too. Maybe it showed up in your love of building things, painting, photography, or that unexplainable thrill of making something yours. I never saw creativity sold as a "career move" thirty years ago, but today, people like Mr. Beast—a YouTuber who built a billion-dollar empire without a degree—prove the rules have changed.

► **PRO-TIP**

Curious how someone with zero academic degrees became the world's richest YouTuber? Look up Mr. Beast's story on the *Diary of a CEO* podcast. His obsession, discipline, and belief in the impossible will make you rethink everything you learned about success.

That's why I didn't flinch when my teenage daughter casually replied, "I wanna be a YouTuber," when I queried what subjects she planned to choose in her final years of high school—the ones that supposedly line you up for a "reputable" university degree. Actually, I almost said, "Good on you!" Instead, I bit my tongue, nodded like a mature adult, and walked away because I knew that if I stuck around, I might start projecting my generational regrets all over her dreams, and that's not the legacy I want to pass on.

Hence, I did what felt safest: I shoved my dreams into the corner, buried them under culture, logic, and loyalty, and told myself that pharmacy school was the smarter choice. And that is how you kill dreams. That's how you stifle creativity and suffocate parts of yourself. When you trade what your heart aches for in exchange for what society applauds. When you let culture, expectations, and a fear of disapproval become the masters of your fate. That's when you lose yourself. And what do you get in return? Applause for being "responsible"!

Part of me still regrets giving up on my dreams. I know that might sound dramatic, but if you've ever shut the door on something that made you come alive, then you get it. I understand where our parents were coming from. They weren't trying to kill our joy; they were simply trying to protect us, to anchor us in certainty. And maybe my dad was right to be cautious, as only a sliver of people make it in the arts. But here's what I think some parents miss: millions have made it to the top without a degree, from authors to media moguls to tech giants. Many started broke, rejected, and unqualified, but they kept going.

When I look back at everything I've achieved in my pharmacy career—nearly two decades of showing up and solving problems—I know that if I'd gone down that path, I would've carried the same fire with me, the same grit. Not because I'm extraordinary, but because chasing what you want most demands a conviction deeper than any job description.

Only years later did the other part of me find comfort in the realization that my degree is a key that opens many doors. Did my pharmacy degree specifically prepare me to write a book? Nope. Did it stop me? Absolutely not. It actually is the launchpad that got me here. It gave me transferable skills that I can apply to any domain. And, most importantly, it taught me to think critically, evaluate situations, and communicate clearly and confidently. These are the skills that stick—the ones you can carry into any room.

A degree in pharmacy gave me the foundation for a promising career, but success, meaning, and purpose were still lacking because I adhered too tightly to the script given to me. I believed I could only practice one way or follow the path others before me had taken. I shut out opportunities because I was too finite-minded and scared. It wasn't until I let go of the script and mustered the courage to explore and purposefully take the Unscripted path that I fulfilled the promise meant for me and found my true calling.

Your job and your current life situation are not preventing you from finding your calling, but the limitations you place on yourself are. The narrative that's replaying in your mind is your worst enemy. On the one hand, you ask yourself, "Is this it?" because you long for fulfillment. On the other hand, you continually silence that voice by answering, "Just be grateful and don't ask for more." You are afraid of stepping out of your comfort zone for fear of failure, fear of what society will think, or because of the burden of family responsibilities. I know this to be true because I faced those same inner demons. But once I went all in on the Unscripted path, that's when I unearthed the potential of what pharmacy has to offer.

You are meant for more. You are allowed to seek it. And you absolutely have what it takes to achieve the fullness of your potential, which is why I wrote this book: to help you realize that your degree does not define you or guarantee you the ultimate fulfillment, joy, and "the more" you are seeking unless you allow it. Only then will you unlock the full potential that lies deep within you.

These are the truths I wish I had known back in 2007, when I pursued pharmacy and felt rejected after not securing an internship.

Unscript Yourself Echoes

The truth that society doesn't tell you.

A degree may allow you to earn more money (sometimes!), but it certainly does not guarantee wealth. And when I say wealth, I'm not only talking about money; I'm talking about the kind of wealth that includes your health, your mental bandwidth, the ability to wake up without a sense of dread, and the freedom to spend time with your family.

When we define wealth by money alone and pursue a degree for financial gain, we end up with disappointment, disillusionment, and that "wanting more but never quite finding it" feeling. And we haven't even talked about joy yet. There are plenty of people who will tell you they're *content* with their degrees. But are they *joyous* about it? That's a different story.

The type of wealth or "joy" you're looking for isn't found in the degree promising you the ultimate freedom; that is the lie that you and I are conditioned to believe. We're told, explicitly and subtly, that this is the summit to climb. That once you arrive, life will finally open its gates to wealth, security, and happiness. What we're rarely taught is that this is an inherited illusion, passed down, polished, and perpetuated by generations who believed in its safety because they had to.

This illusion doesn't shout. It hums quietly beneath school desks and in the pride of graduation speeches. It's reinforced by brochures, career fairs, and the applause of our well-meaning parents. And so we follow the path. We blindly comply and stretch ourselves thin as we chase the credentials we believed would be meaningful, only to arrive and feel the ache of disillusionment.

A degree opens the door, but it is not synonymous with freedom. Freedom is not something handed to you by an institution; it's something built from within, slowly, often painfully, when you question the blueprint you were handed. When that silent ache starts to creep in, and your inner voice gets louder, asking, *Is this it?* That's when it finally hits you like a freight train: *Did I take the right path?*

Now, don't get me wrong. I'm not here to bash pharmacy, education, or ambition. There is absolutely nothing wrong with external achievements, with having a good societal reputation and earning degrees; that isn't the point of this book. What I am saying is that your degree is not the destination. It's the departure point. It might define the shape of your career. It might (unfortunately) become society's shortcut for determining your worth. But you must never let it define your identity or your destination. A degree provides you with a stable job that earns you money, but it doesn't define your worth or your destiny.

Faith Echoes

God doesn't give you talents to shelve them.

There is a sacred-sounding lie that floats through every healthcare profession: *If you're not suffering or sacrificing something, then it must not be holy.*

But here's the truth no one preaches loudly enough: God doesn't give us talents to shelve them for practicality. He doesn't call us to martyr our gifts on the altar of stability; He calls us to steward them. Your creativity, your love of beauty, and your desire to write, speak, or build something new are not selfish. That's your calling. Here I am using my talent for creative writing to serve you, and God wants the same for each of you.

Scripture says, "Each of you should use whatever gift you have received to serve others" (1 Peter 4:10). That doesn't mean we all have to serve the same way. You can be called to pharmacy and still be called to *more.* You can pay the bills and still write poetry. You can serve patients and still honor the storyteller, the artist, and the singer inside you. Don't confuse service with silence and mistake duty for your whole destiny.

Unscript Yourself Toolkit

Permission to Want More Again

Come as you are. Skip perfection.
One heartfelt line per prompt is better than ten perfect ones.

What dreams have you buried—the ones you rarely admit, even to yourself?

___
___
___

What talents have you pushed to the sidelines instead of treating them as gifts worth nurturing?

___
___
___

What fears are holding you back from pursuing the "more" you feel called to—whether in pharmacy, a creative project, or a path outside your degree?

___
___
___

If you gave yourself permission to revive one of those dreams or talents, what small first step could you take this month?

___
___
___

Unscripted Affirmation

My dreams have not passed me by. They are waiting. I am allowed to want more than the script I was handed.

CHAPTER 2

You Are Not Meant to Fit the Mold

Rejection is redirection.

—Bryant McGill

I never fit the mold. I first slammed into that truth in my first year of university when it became painfully evident that the system was rigid and I was not, and no matter how hard I tried to contort myself into its shape, it would never call that a strength. Being schooled by a system that prized compliance over curiosity slowly left me feeling rejected and worn down. And if you've felt that friction, too, know that it isn't failure; it's information that will arm you with the confidence to go on the Unscripted path. On Purpose.

I made it through the academic hoops of the foundation pre-pharmacy year and began my Bachelor of Pharmacy journey in 2004. But while I was accepted on paper, I felt rejected by the culture.

The city I studied in was infamous back then for beer-fueled rites of passage—couches set ablaze and tossed into the river like sacrifices to adolescent chaos. So, campus life was split into two species: front-row sitters speaking in molecular structures, and the weekend crowd who made sacrifices at four a.m. I wasn't either. I existed in the blur between them. And in that in-between space, when you don't feel you belong anywhere, your mental health begins to unravel quietly, and you gaslight yourself by thinking, *It's all in your head.*

I'm sure you've had such times in your life when you've numbed your pain by overworking or studying, so I buried my head in my books and attempted to find comfort in the stuff-it-in-your-brain-then-vomit-it-on-paper approach to learning. Some of us are more curiosity-led, hands-on learners—the kind who ask why until someone gives up trying to answer. I am one of those. Though I struggled, I performed well on paper; numbers didn't betray me even when my spirit was running on fumes. There was a flatness to the experience, as if I were being asked to study color through grayscale slides. Years later, a personality profile finally named it: I'm a creative, tactile learner—someone who needs to talk, explore, and connect. No wonder I felt like I was drowning in a sea of academic sterility.

Despite that, I kept going. Sometimes turning around feels impossible. I was haunted by what everyone at school would think of me. I also feared letting my parents down, failing in society, and the uncertainty of what else I could do with my life. Everyone around me stayed the course, so surely something was wrong with me. *Follow the crowd, Katrina!* was the phrase that played on a loop inside my head more often than I would've liked. And sometimes, if I were lucky, a softer murmur would follow: *It'll get better. You'll find yourself in this.* And gratefully, I did. Eventually. As in fifteen years later. Hopefully, this won't be your timeline because you're here, reading this!

And I can say this now: neither you nor I were created to fit in, and why would we try to? Life would be boring if we were all the same. Those sleepless nights, those mysterious headaches, and that internal conflict are there to tell you something important: you are meant for more and to push you to seek it. Only years later—after peeling back the layers and learning to listen to my nervous system after it crashed—did I realize it wasn't burnout. It was misalignment. Profound, disorienting misalignment. And you know how exhausting it is to carry so much uncertainty while pretending convincingly to be fine. Misalignment between how I'm built and the societal structures I kept trying to live inside.

So, back to the beginning. It was now halfway through my final year of pharmacy school, and everyone had secured their internship (a practical year that every graduating pharmacy student must complete before they register as a pharmacist). I was confident that I had secured mine. The pharmacy I worked at during the summer breaks assured me they would accept me as an intern. Well, with a change of management, they changed their minds. They told me this after most internship sites across the country had been secured. I felt devastated. All I wanted after surviving burning couches was to be back in my hometown.

I frantically started looking for positions, even in rural areas, but received rejection letter after another. Those who have experienced rejection will be familiar with those templated "We regret to inform you" emails that take your inbox by storm. I received so many that I considered binding them into a rejection anthology titled *Regretfully Declined: A Pharmacist's Guide to Rejection.*

One of the most bizarre rejections I'll never forget was a phone call that went something like this: "I actually don't know why I am declining you. Your interview went pretty well. I guess, and I don't know how to put it, but you came across as extremely persistent, which isn't necessarily a bad thing." At the time, those words broke me. I remember hanging up and staring blankly at the wall, wondering if I'd somehow misunderstood the definition of the word *persistence.* Since when was persistence a flaw? It felt like someone had looked at my strength—the fuel that had kept me upright through academic misery and emotional fog—and labeled it a liability.

And here's the cruel yet beautiful twist: that same persistence, the trait that made me "too much" in that moment, is what carried me through the years to come. It's what helped me keep questioning, keep searching, and keep *becoming.* That offhand rejection taught me that no one will ever see your hidden potential the way you can. The very traits that make you come alive are often misread or dismissed when you're trying to fit into someone else's mold. And that's because you're not meant to. If you've been told your persistence is "too much," or "you're not the right fit," translate those words to mean: "I don't know what to do with your drive." Rejection stings, yes, but it's also data. Rejection isn't saying, "You're not enough," but "You're not right for this room."

So if something good in your character reads as a flaw, you're in the wrong room, and throughout this book, I'll show you how I built my own room.

The very traits that make you come alive are often misread or dismissed when you're trying to fit into someone else's mold.

During these times of rejection, no matter how much you push yourself to keep going, it's normal to question everything—your path, your choices, and even yourself. It feels like a slap in the face. The "you're not good enough" vibes linger for months afterward. They burrow in and play on your insecurities. And so, my self-esteem hit rock bottom. *Maybe this was never meant to be for me* became my mantra. *Maybe I should've chased my creative talents.* Every night, I'd fold my hands in quiet desperation: *Please, God, I've had enough. You know I've worked so hard this year. You know how lonely it's been. You promised You had plans for me, plans to prosper me, to give me hope and a future.* But it was as though my prayers hit a brick wall. It felt like I was lobbing desperate words into an empty sky, as if God had put me on hold.

Little did I know then that *rejection is redirection.* That the right opportunity that will shape your life and character will come. The rejections are there to channel you to the path you are destined for. Saying, "I am so grateful for the rejections" would be an understatement because, without them, I wouldn't be here. I wouldn't be writing this book, which, if I'm being honest, feels more aligned with my soul's work than any job I've held before. This feeling of fulfillment comes when you accept rejection and let go of the script.

When everything seemed to collapse, I found myself sitting across from the associate dean of the pharmacy school, pleading for

► **REFLECTION**

When have you mistaken divine silence for divine absence? What were you being prepared for in that waiting season? Looking back, was it really silence, or did God have something better on hold for you?

► **PRO-TIP**

If you're stuck without a job offer, don't be afraid to ask for help. Pride won't pay your bills, but courage might.

help. To this day, I remain deeply grateful that she looked out for me, kept an eye on roles as they opened up, and offered the one thing I needed most in that moment: a sliver of hope, because she knew how hardworking I was. This is where I'll pause and say: work hard (and smart!), not to please people, but because when you do that, life will reward you by sending people to help you at every step of the journey. The world calls it karma; I call it divine intervention.

It wasn't until I was completing the end-of-year exams that a pharmacy proprietor from a small rural pharmacy in the North Island of the country reached out to request a face-to-face interview. I was so homesick that the very thought of living somewhere so remote, with no familiar faces or rhythms of home, was almost enough to make me quit pharmacy altogether. I finished my Friday exam and flew up for the interview. I was accepted for the position, and frankly, it felt like mutual desperation.

"Can we sign a contract?" I blurted out, clinging to the one lifeline I had in that moment. I was heading overseas that summer for my wedding, and the owner reassured me, "No, have your wedding, and we'll sign it when you start in February."

I'm sure you've probably sat in your own milestone moment, feeling the ache under the joy, and that's exactly what I was feeling in that moment—happiness blended with despair. I was meant to be celebrating one of the most significant milestones of my life, yet there was a heaviness I couldn't shake—a knowing that I was walking toward something I *really* didn't want.

What happened next was nothing short of a miracle, or a misfortune in disguise. While it cracked me open, it also carved me into someone who could withstand the hardships to come. It shaped the core of who I am today—and yes, it is another rejection but of a different kind.

Unscript Yourself Echoes

Rejection gives you permission to build your own mold.

The rejection of others is not a verdict on your worth. Sometimes it is purely logistical, such as when there are multiple exceptional candidates. Sometimes it is a fit of values and strategy. And rarely, it can represent a threat. Not a threat of who you are, but of what you represent: success, possibility, boldness. In those moments, it can feel like you're being pushed away because your presence invites a reckoning someone isn't ready to face. This doesn't mean the rejection won't ache, and the goal isn't to numb the pain but to reframe the meaning: "This door closed so the one meant for me can open."

If you reflect on your life, you will see that every door that closed opened better doors. Yet I completely understand how this feels for those who are early in the journey. The way through is to allow yourself to sit with the pain of rejection. You are human, after all. Then you must review your application and ask for specific feedback from a trusted mentor or colleague. When you do so, you will return to the application process with clarity and alignment.

Faith Echoes

It's better to want what's good in the long run than what's good now.

Sometimes the doors that slam shut are a mercy in disguise. The rejections, the diversions, the abrupt endings are not punishments but protection. Can you think of a moment you thought was the end, only to realize later it was the redirection you needed?

And here's what's more profound: In seasons like this, when all we get back from God is silence, when our faith feels paper-thin, and when we wonder if God is really there, it's easy to become short-sighted. To want what appears good now, not what is good in the long run.

Only eighteen years later, when I look back, do I realize how amazing God is. Only now do I see how wildly good God has been to me. How that silence wasn't abandonment; it was acknowledgment. How the rejection was a disguised blessing. How the waiting didn't crush me; it cracked me open in the best possible way. Sometimes I wish an apology could reach God—one that says, *I'm sorry for doubting You. I'm sorry for thinking You had forgotten me.* But I know He doesn't need my guilt; He wants my trust. And this became the best testing ground for my faith.

Romans 8:28: *"And we know that in all things God works for the good of those who love him, who have been called according to his purpose."*

Jeremiah 29:11: *"For I know the plans I have for you," declares the LORD, "plans to prosper you and not to harm you, plans to give you hope and a future."*

Unscript Yourself Toolkit

Permission to Build Your Own Room

Bring your honest self. One messy truth is worth more than polished silence.

Think of a time you were rejected. How did it make you feel? Fast-forward a few years: What doors closed? What doors opened? Which "too much" trait actually helped you get to where you are now?

____

____

____

If you're in that season now: What data is this "no" giving you about the room (not you)? What is one step you can take to turn it around?

____

____

____

Unscripted Permission Slips

- Embrace rejection. Treat it as data that points you to the path you're meant to be on.
- If your drive and persistence are treated as flaws, then it's the wrong room. And if no room fits, it's time to build one yourself.
- You have permission to ask for help before you break. Growth happens with support over secrecy.

Unscripted Affirmation

I am not meant to fit in. I am created on purpose, for a purpose. If I can't find it in a prebuilt room, then I have permission to build my own.

PART II

The Crucible

"The world has so many lessons to teach you. These lessons often come dressed up as detours or roadblocks, and if you get the lesson, you pass, and if you don't, you have to repeat the class. The lesson will keep showing up until you learn it."

—OPRAH WINFREY

CHAPTER 3

You Are Allowed to Pause When Rejection Hurts

The pain you feel today
will be the strength you feel tomorrow.
—Ritu Ghatourey

After four years of struggling to fit into a culture I failed to belong to, the idea of retreating further into professional isolation felt less like a noble calling and more like voluntary exile. But I could see there was space to grow, an opportunity to serve, and a desperate need for patient care in rural areas. Because here is what I didn't know early in my career: it is much easier to climb the ladder, gain diverse experience, and grow in a smaller workplace.

Some situations test your faith and values, such as layoffs, career detours that don't go your way, and colleagues who test your boundaries, among other things. And though we know that there is a lesson to learn from it all, embracing and accepting the disappointments in the moment is something we wrestle with. Despite that, I told myself I could survive it. No matter how lonely, how silent, how soul-dampening that year might be, I'd grit my teeth and get through. What harm would one more year of self-sacrifice do if it meant staying in the game?

So I rehearsed my acceptance—the kind when you whisper prayers through clenched teeth: *God, thank You. But also, I'm angry, and I'm not feeling grateful, except maybe I am.* And as you pray, you're not sure if you are surrendering or settling because you know He is good. You trust Him, but you're not feeling it right away.

Here is what bothers me about that situation from a pharmacy leader's perspective: If someone like me, who deeply cares about access and equity, still couldn't say yes to rural practice, what hope is there for pharmacist retention? And I hated what that said about me. Though I accepted the role, I carried this quiet, shame-soaked guilt for not wanting it. It felt like I was turning my back on a community that deserved better, like I was betraying my own values around service, justice, and showing up where it matters.

Anyhow, it was 3:20 a.m. on some unremarkable day in November 2007, when a tiny sliver of hope slid into my inbox—an email from someone on the Pharmaceutical Society's internship team. Sleep was a scarce commodity for me during that time, and something inside me said a better opportunity was coming and that I should not give up hope.

Despite the inner positivity, anxiety gets hold of us—that split-second gut-wrench when you're waiting on news, when your inbox pings, and your whole body flinches. It's a cocktail of hope and dread. I hovered over the email, half-wanting to open it, half-dreading what it might confirm. I expected the usual letdown: another sorry-we-tried-but-no-luck message. But it was some positive news . . . at last! The email stated that a pharmacist in Christchurch (my city!) was actively seeking an intern, had received my CV, and wanted to interview me. I blinked and reread it to be sure I wasn't hallucinating from lack of sleep.

Before my brain had the chance to catch up, my fingers were already firing off a reply. I introduced myself, expressed my keenest interests, and politely begged for a Skype interview because I was overseas—thank God for technology! And yes, I'm fully

► **PRO-TIP**

I won't spiral into a systems rant (though my inner strategist is twitching), but I'll say this: If we are serious about solving pharmacy deserts, we need to embrace models that allow remote pharmacists to serve communities via depot-style medication hubs (sneaking this one in here in case an advocacy leader is reading and feeling Unscripted enough to run with it.)

cringing, remembering that this was back in the era of clunky webcams and dial-up speeds—the days when opening Skype required patience usually reserved for sainthood. There I was, blinking into a fuzzy webcam, being grilled on insulin dose calculations while my already overloaded brain struggled to keep pace.

► **REFLECTION**

When was the last time you almost gave up only to have something shift at the final hour? What would you say now to the version of you that was hanging on by a thread?

That's when I heard my favorite concluding sentence: "We'll get back to you." And, of course, I knew what that meant. Any pharmacist reading this knows the code. "We'll be in touch" is a polite way of saying, "Don't call us; we'll ghost you." This seems like the appropriate place to insert my plea to pharmacy proprietors and any pharmacy HR personnel reading this, because someone needs to say it: If you decline an applicant, at least provide them with pointers on areas for improvement. Your guidance could change their career because they won't know where to improve unless someone tells them.

I left that interview so heavy-hearted. You can feel it in your bones when an interview has gone off the rails. No amount of post-call pep talks can drown out the gnawing certainty that you didn't only miss the mark; you never even saw the target. If I'm honest, I didn't prepare for that interview because I didn't think it would go anywhere. I'd had so many dead ends that any signs of hope felt dangerous. And when the interview finally came, I was caught between wanting it so badly I could barely breathe and not trusting it enough to show up fully. That's the thing about rejection fatigue: It doesn't just make you tired; it makes you sabotage the very thing you once prayed for and screw it up.

And I knew the moment I clicked that Godforsaken red button to hang up that what I had brought into that interview wasn't confidence, clarity, or coherence. It was pure, undiluted desperation. The kind that makes your voice tremble in places you didn't think nerves could reach and turns your words into scattered gravel instead of sentences. Recalling the interview, I tried to impress with the usual song—*Look how excellent my grades are!*—but had nothing real to show for it in terms of my problem-solving skills or actual contributions. Never mind the fact that I'd worked in a pharmacy every summer, or that I had a natural way with patients, or that I'd delivered five-star service and topped the sales scoreboards. None of that came through. Instead, all I portrayed was a frantic energy that screamed, "Please accept me!" louder than any actual skill ever could.

Later, with the clarity that only hindsight and a bruised ego can provide, I came to realize something that wasn't covered in pharmacy school: employers don't like desperation. At all. If you've been tracking with me through the last chapters, you'll remember my earlier lesson about the employer who called me out on my "persistence" being the issue, but it wasn't persistence. It was desperation. There's a difference. A desperate spirit leaks into the room before you speak. It clings to your voice, your posture, and the energy behind your carefully rehearsed answers. It whispers: *I need out.* Not, *I believe I'm a good fit*, but *Please, rescue me.* And here's the kicker: desperation doesn't make people want to help you. It makes them wonder what you're running from. And that's never a good sign. Because if you've run away from other employers, you'll likely run away from them, too.

This was the interview that taught me how to show up in interviews. No matter how desperate I might feel to escape my current circumstances, I owe it to myself and to the person on the other side to separate my panic from my pitch. To bring forward not just my list of qualifications but real, tangible examples of how I've solved problems, contributed to growth, and delivered value. Because that's what employers want: your discernment and your ability to translate experience into future impact.

Of course, clarity doesn't erase disappointment. So I went through the five stages of grief and came to accept my fate: I had just bombed an opportunity to escape what I was sure would be a year of pure misery. So I did what any semi-functional adult in emotional survival mode does: I clung to the lessons learned, slapped on some forced gratitude, and convinced myself I should be thankful I had a position and that a door had opened at all.

It was a few days later, while I was mentally preparing for my departure into the unknown world of rural pharmacy and browsing flats to rent, that a response arrived

► **PRO-TIP**

Never walk into an interview carrying desperation. Leave it at the door. Take with you your value and proof of what you've brought to the table in the past, such as examples of your projects or successes. Let the evidence of your past impact speak for itself.

in my inbox. I sat there, eyes glued to the subject line. It might as well have said, "This will determine if you're enough." So, with a pounding heart and clammy palms, I opened that email. My eyes frantically scanned the first line for the usual bureaucratic heartbreak—those tidy rejection clichés—and when they didn't appear, the air came back into my lungs. I got the position.

But the strangest thing happened. Relief didn't flood in like I'd imagined it would. Instead, I felt this muted exhale, like the body's response to narrowly escaping a car crash. If you've ever had many things not go your way, you'll relate to that feeling when you want to be happy, but somehow you can't get yourself to be. I felt so numb from all the past rejections that I couldn't accept the new reality. Gratitude was present, yes, but so was exhaustion and a gnawing unease that I couldn't quite name.

I wish I could write that everything changed after I got the job offer; that the long nights and the bruised faith all melted away into something smooth and celebratory. But I won't lie to you. That year was a crucible. It was the kind of year that didn't just test you—it tore you open and asked, "*What are you really made of?*" The kind that reveals whether your faith is performative or real. It was the year that slowly, methodically stripped away all my illusions about what it meant to "make it" as a pharmacist.

I responded to the offer with immense gratitude (but with less desperate energy this time). And, of course, I asked about signing a contract, which he sent without delay because I wasn't going to risk waiting.

But here's the twist: If I had signed a contract with that rural pharmacy, the one for which I had been interviewed a couple of months earlier, I couldn't have withdrawn and accepted this offer. This is where I think fate (I call it God) works in the most astonishing ways. Ways beyond our comprehension. Ways that make no sense while you're sitting there in the middle of the wreckage. Only later can you trace the path backward and see there was a design all along. God knows and owns the future. He already had it all laid out in a plan. I wish I'd trusted Him more.

Some days of my internship year felt like redemption, and others felt like punishment. But this I'm certain of: I wouldn't erase any of the experiences I gained—not a single day, not the hardest shift. Because that year built something in me that ease never could. It gave me calluses in the places I used to bleed. It taught me that getting what you prayed for doesn't mean the storm is over; it means you're now officially an attendee in Earth school, and you're going to have to pass the exam.

Unscript Yourself Echoes

Rejection is an opportunity for pause and realignment.

The thing we don't do enough of is allow ourselves to feel the ache of rejection, the sting of shame, or the slow erosion of not being chosen. And I say *we* because I've been there. It's almost like there's an unspoken agreement in healthcare: pretend the pain didn't happen, keep moving, stay productive, bury the bruise beneath the white coat, and call it resilience. And a brain that echoes, *If you're going to show up for patients, you've got to have it all together.*

But you know what that does?

It short-circuits the learning. It silences the questions that might've led us somewhere useful. It doesn't give us space to ask: *Where did I go wrong? What actually worked? What might I do differently next time if I dared to slow down long enough to look honestly at the wreckage?*

Instead, we "panic-apply." We shotgun our CVs into the void and show up for interviews as if we're on life support. And in the rush, we forget things, like changing the name on the cover letter. (If you've done that, I see you because I've done it too. No, it wasn't a good look, and yes, the shame still lingers.)

Then the rejection comes, or worse, the silence. We hate that feeling so much that we sprint to fill out the next application. We move on fast—too fast—without pause or reflection. Without allowing ourselves to sit with the rejection and the shame, to process it and heal from it because it feels so heavy, we can't bear to hold it. In fact, we're ashamed that we feel ashamed, so we suppress it, slap on a professional face, and march on as if it didn't gut us. But that doesn't make the pain go away. It leaks out later, usually as desperation, which we carry into the next interview like invisible static. Desperation that clings to our voice, stiffens our posture, and sends off quiet alarm bells to the person across the desk. They might not name it, but they can feel it. And it doesn't read as passion; it reads as panic.

We forget the human beneath the white coat—that we're allowed to counsel others through heartbreak while still nursing our own. But when we fail to acknowledge our wounds, when we pretend to have it all together, we end up bleeding anyway, but in places no one can see, not even ourselves. And here's the kicker: Employers not only read your CV; they read your spirit. They read the energy behind your words and the story behind your sentences. And when desperation replaces discernment, it repels the very thing you're chasing.

So before you apply, before you show up, before you rehearse the perfect answer to "tell me about yourself," ask yourself this: *"Am I reaching for this because it's aligned, or because I'm drowning and need something (anything) to pull me to shore?"*

If the only reason you want the role is that it gets you out of your misery by Christmas, that's drowning. If you're drowning, please take the time to sit with the rejection and absorb its sting before applying for more jobs. As I reflect on the times I was rejected, even though it was God's plan, I firmly believe I carried such desperate energy into my communications, both in person and via email, that it was detected and led to further rejections. Don't be me!

Faith Echoes

God desires your honest prayers, not your polished ones.

Have you ever whispered a prayer that felt more like a protest? One of those moments when you thank God through clenched teeth, not because you're ungrateful, but because gratitude feels like a betrayal of your pain? You know, those prayers when the words come out wrapped in anger and aching trust all at once? These are the sacred tensions where faith gets real. They are not polished prayers but honest prayers that we pray while barely holding on. So pause and ask: *What's one moment in my life when I wanted to trust but also walk away? And what did I do with that ache?*

God understands our weakness. He gets our anger in these moments.

And He wants us to take that to Him rather than keep our pain silent. These are the moments when He wants us to reach out and plead to Him, like the father who reached out to Him to heal his son, who was suffering from a deaf and mute spirit, saying:

"I believe; help my unbelief!" Mark 9:24 (ESV).

Because life is but a test of our faith, it is these moments that define and strengthen it. If we only experienced positive outcomes, we would not hold onto our faith.

Unscript Yourself Toolkit

Permission to Pause for Alignment

Show up with your coffee, your chaos, and your authentic self. A single raw line can shift more than a polished paragraph.

Where in your life do you feel rejection fatigue creeping in?

____

____

____

What is one way you can pause without guilt before you jump into the following application, project, or commitment?

____

____

____

What "muted wins" have you brushed past without celebrating? How might you honor them this week?

____

____

____

Unscripted Permission Slips

- You have permission to feel tired without being "weak."
- You have permission to pray angry prayers and still call it faith.
- You have permission to stop panic-applying and seek alignment instead.

Unscripted Affirmation

Rejection does not define me. I can pause, I can ache, and I can rise without apology.

CHAPTER 4

You Are Not Your Mistakes

Your mistakes don't define you. It's your reaction to the mistake that defines you.

—Katrina Azer

My internship began in February 2008, and it was filled with such chaos that it made me question my existence while simultaneously challenging me to become the best version of myself.

Life sometimes tests you through people; you know, the ones you mutter about under your breath in the moment and end up thanking for the grit they gave you. That's how I felt about my preceptor. He spotted glimpses of promise in me and wanted to fast-track me into the pharmacist he knew I could become. But he was tough—a "you'll thank me one day" kind of tough. He demanded precision, speed, and confidence—qualities I had not yet grown into but was expected to perform as though I had.

Sometimes he'd ask me clinical questions that only an experienced pharmacist would answer without breaking a sweat. In those moments, I wished he would extend a hand, but his method rarely changed: "Find the answer yourself." I resented it then, but I am grateful for it now. Because later, when the dispensary turned to smoke, when the phones screamed, and the scripts arrived bristling with clinical knots while patients waited, I didn't flinch. I trusted myself to hunt the truth in real time. I was thrown into the deep end from day one.

I do not doubt that you'll have some experiences in your career that have shaped you more than your degree ever did. I know this because now I am reminded of the highlights, the mishaps, and the drastic errors that shaped me more than any textbook ever did.

And in those times, I wish I had dared to say, "I'm not okay." But when your license feels like a ticking bomb you're barely qualified to carry, there's no room for honesty. You don't correct the person in charge or admit that the pressure is getting to you. And so I did what so many early-career pharmacists do: I swallowed my fear, cinched my silence tight around my throat, and learned to endure.

For starters, I hated—viscerally—the dissonance between what I was taught at university and what I was actually doing behind the counter. I had studied for clinical impact. But, of course, when you're the trainee, you're the designated understudy for every unpopular task. So, I got stuck in a cramped corner of the dispensary every single day, packing medication blisters—a mind-numbing ritual of robotic fingers and color-coded compartments. But boredom can be its own boot camp. Just as every pharmacist does, I learned what medications looked like. I could tell you the difference between amlodipine and atenolol in my sleep. Little did I know that obsessive familiarity would one day become my secret weapon. It made me a Michelin-meticulous checking pharmacist.

Though the total lack of patient interaction during those first few months grated on me, I had signed up to help people—to connect, to consult, to be part of someone's healing. But instead, my neurons fired in constant revolt: *Is this what you signed up for, for the rest of your life?* The dread crept in like fog, thick and unshakable. I remember standing by the counter one day, checking expiry dates while my insides screamed. And yet, I said nothing.

I silenced the voice and convinced myself it was just the training year and that things would get better. *They had to.*

In hindsight, I'm glad I had those experiences. Not because they felt good, but because they taught me how to embrace the thankless tasks without losing myself to bitterness. If there's one principle that's carried me far in pharmacy and life, it's this: Do the work no one else wants to do. Do it excellently, quietly, and without performative martyrdom. You'll learn faster. You'll stand out, and eventually, if the system is half-way decent, you'll rise high enough to choose what you take on.

► PRO-TIP

If you want to stand out, do the work rejected by others. Pharmacy residencies and early-career years often involve menial tasks, but those who master the mundane tasks build real clinical and professional stamina that future-proofs their careers. Character is forged in the corners.

As the months went on, I got to know more of my patients by their drug charts and their stories. I got to know their routines, their lives, and their heartbreaks. You even get to know their dogs' names. *(I'm always amazed by the details patients share with their community pharmacist!)*

That's what makes me believe that pharmacists have a golden, sacred opportunity that no AI or clinical algorithm can replicate. It lies in the depths of the human connection we build with our patients. We are, after all, the health professionals seen most often. And no matter what technology does to this profession—no matter what tasks get automated or delegated—the relationship, the rapport, and the sacred familiarity are what we must keep alive.

Back to my life as a trainee pharmacist: I was not winning any awards in the dispensing department. In fact, I was a terrible dispensing pharmacist. It still brings me a deep, stomach-tightening shame to this day because I wasn't just making mistakes; I was making them on repeat. Not because I didn't care, but because I hadn't built a deep understanding of the weight of what a dispensing error could cost. There were times when the wrong drug, the wrong strength, or the wrong label nearly made its way into someone's home. While every one of those mistakes was caught before it left the dispensary, they didn't escape my preceptor's attention. He pulled me aside and told me to slow down and pay attention. I always nodded and apologized, but I still didn't change.

Looking back, I can finally name what was happening to me. I wasn't careless; I was disconnected. I hated the monotony of the

---

Near-miss/mistake: an error that was caught *before* causing harm, during the checking process, and before the patient receives the prescription.

Dispensing error: an error detected *after* the patient receives the prescription.

dispensing process. My neurodivergent brain was hungry for complexity, constantly scanning for novelty, and I couldn't tolerate the sheer predictability of those tasks. No one warned me that the majority of my day would be spent counting pills. I didn't know how to override the mental resistance I felt toward such tasks without sounding entitled..

The near-misses weren't just sloppy errors but symptoms of misalignment between what I thought I had signed up for and what I was actually doing day after day. They were a manifestation of quiet frustration, creative claustrophobia, and disillusionment so deep I hadn't yet found the courage to admit it. And maybe you have had a moment like that too—when you stared down a never-ending queue of prescriptions to be dispensed and thought, *This wasn't the deal. This isn't why I sacrificed so much.*

Let me make this clear: Dispensing is not the enemy. Counting, checking, and preparing medicines are necessary, sacred parts of the work, and someone has to do them with care. For some pharmacists, that rhythm of the bench is its own kind of sanctuary, and if that's you, please know that it is holy work I deeply respect. But I came to accept that dispensing alone was no longer my gateway to serving patients well; I loved being at the front counter with patients, but the endless counting in fives slowly hollowed me out in a way I could no longer ignore.

Unfortunately for me, that misalignment culminated in precisely what you'd expect: patient harm and a lesson that changed my career trajectory.

One afternoon, a woman slid a pillbox across the counter and said, "I've been taking these pills. They look different from my usual ones. I thought it was a brand change, but I started feeling light-headed and got headaches I couldn't shake. Can you check them?"

My heart pounded. My first instinct was to have my preceptor handle it, but he was on leave. I had been under the supervision of a locum pharmacist for two weeks. That meant I had to deal with this complaint. I, the woefully inexperienced trainee pharmacist, was now the only "regular" on-site, and a patient was depending on *me* to fix the problem. I stared at the box. The medication's name stared back. I secretly prayed it might've been the locum who handled that particular script, but I knew it was me. Desperation made me dig deeper, so

I marched to the script records and started hunting, my heart lodged in my throat. Suddenly, the gut-wrenching "oh no" moment arrived—the kind that makes time slow down and your breath stop. Yep, I had screwed up big time and dispensed dothiepin (dosulepin) 75 mg instead of doxepin 25 mg.

My career felt like dust slipping through my fingers. The weight of what I had done hit me with full force, like a freight train of shame. What's worse is that I had zero training on how to handle it. What do you actually say when you've made a mistake that adversely impacts someone's health? How do you reassure the patient without inflaming the situation? How do you inform the patient of their rights without sounding legalistic or cold? I wished, then, that pharmacy school had drilled us not only in pharmacodynamics but also in human dynamics, especially when things go sideways.

I took the box over to the locum pharmacist. My legs felt like cement. She scanned the label, saw her checking initials scrawled beside mine, and without a word of judgment or blame, took over. She stepped into the lead, managing the situation calmly. I stood beside her, equal parts relieved and sick to my stomach. I was relieved that for a brief, flickering moment, I was not the *only* one responsible. But I was nauseated by the knowledge that a human being had suffered discomfort, dizziness, and who knows what else because of a mistake that *I* had made. The locum's signature might have been on the label, but the fingerprints were mine. In fairness, she likely caught a dozen other mistakes I made that week, and this one simply slipped through the cracks.

I stood there, rooted to the same square of floor tiles, and my instinct screamed to excuse myself and retreat into the staff toilet and let the walls catch my panic. But a voice inside me whispered, *You don't get to run. Not this time. You made this mess. You're going to stand here and learn how to manage it.* So I stayed, listened, and learned how to be present in the aftermath of harm—how to hold space for the discomfort I had caused.

She calmly acknowledged the mix-up and explained that the medication names were, unfortunately, confusingly similar in both spelling and therapeutic class. I stood behind her like a ghost of guilt, watching the moment I'd dreaded unfold. I waited for the patient's response and realized that while the world hadn't collapsed, something in me had. Gratefully, she didn't yell or demand a formal complaint process; she was less concerned about the headaches and dizzy spells than she was about simply being on the right medication from now on.

Maybe it helped that the locum gently said, *"Katrina is a trainee pharmacist. She's still learning."* And there it was—that word—*learning.*

So, lesson learned? More like a lesson seared into the folds of my brain so deeply that I can still feel it burn. I was deeply grateful to God that when the lesson finally turned up, it didn't show up wielding heavy armor. No hospital admission, cardiac arrest, or death. Just a wake-up call dressed in a formal suit. *This could've been so much worse,* echoed in my mind like a sacred refrain all night. I prayed, trembling, and asked God—begged Him—to make this the last dispensing error I would ever make. And I'm glad to tell you it was.

That night, I couldn't sleep. At around 2 a.m., I flicked on the harsh fluorescent light of the bathroom and stared into the mirror. Through gritted teeth and half-choked shame, I said, "*If you can't get your bloody act together, then leave pharmacy before you cause irreversible harm.*"

Some may read that and think I was being dramatic, that I was catastrophizing, but the truth was that I was dangerously disconnected from the stakes and the patient on the other side of the counter. If I had kept going like that, if this mistake hadn't shaken me awake, I would have caused irreversible, life-altering, reputation-obliterating harm. And isn't this every pharmacist's worst fear?

The next morning, I walked into work with a churning gut. I prayed for clarity and courage to face my preceptor. I figured it was better he heard it from me than from the dreaded *Interventions and Errors* book, more like the *Book of Sins and Confessions.* Okay, technically it's the "Quality Improvement" log, where you document near-misses and errors so the team can identify trends and reduce future risk. I've never worked in a pharmacy where people liked that book. Most see it as a name-and-shame file dressed up in quality and safety language. And who could blame them? Nobody volunteers to be told they've messed up or wakes up hoping their mistake gets immortalized in ink and logged for audit.

I pulled myself together and broke the dreaded news while trying to be wise in my word choice. I explained that I had made a dispensing error and that the script had left the pharmacy. The patient had taken the medicine and hadn't felt their best. Then I did what all guilty kids do when they're standing at the edge of consequence: I bent my head and looked down at the benchtop like it might somehow save me because I couldn't dare look at him.

There was a long moment of silence. The kind that, despite having no vibrational frequency, still finds a way to crawl through your bones and settle under your skin. His face turned red, understandably, and he said nothing. If only the counting tray had been a portkey. You know, like in the Harry Potter books? Touch it, and *whoosh*, I'm gone. Teleported anywhere else. My head was a swarm of catastrophic predictions: termination, formal reports, internship revoked. Even I was so fed up with my mistakes that I might have welcomed the relief of being told I didn't belong.

Finally, after what felt like a decade of punishment, he asked me to reflect, not just to apologize and move on. He told me that someone's life—and my entire career—was at stake, as if I hadn't already played those thoughts on repeat the whole night. Even so, I needed the pressing reminder. In that moment, I realized something important: this wasn't just about dispensing safely; this was about deciding whether I wanted to be a pharmacist who could be trusted with a life.

So that night, I stayed up in an exhausting bout of introspection and found answers hidden beneath layers of performance-mode survival. I admitted to my unintentional carelessness in an emotionally bankrupt, spiritually absent way, and the shame hit me like a biblical flood. I had been selfish. I had prioritized my feelings about my job—my boredom, my frustration, my silent rebellion—over patient safety.

I realized with unwelcome clarity that my attitude wasn't serving me. Though I disliked my job and resented the system, I was not allowed, under any circumstances, to compromise patient safety; something had to shift radically.

So, I disconnected my logical brain from my emotions and began treating my dispensing shift as sacred ground. The moment I stepped behind that counter, my mood, my burnout, and my frustration got checked at the door. From that moment on, I was there *for them*. Not for me. Not for my personal fulfillment, but for the patient. Because the day you forget what's at stake is the day you become a danger to your patients.

That reflection opened a door I hadn't known was there. One that led me to the *emotional burden* of being a pharmacist. We are the gatekeepers. The final sign-off. The last pair of eyes between human suffering and a potentially catastrophic error. Doctors make errors too, but most of the time, we are the ones who catch them. So when we're the ones who err, who catches us? No one. Only if the patient brings it to our attention, and oftentimes it's too late. We are the end of the line. And that should keep us awake, not with fear but with reverence and gratitude that we get to be entrusted with someone's life.

We are the end of the line. And that should keep us awake, not with fear but with reverence and gratitude that we get to be entrusted with someone's life.

One afternoon, while flipping through my internship folder to complete yet another assignment, I spotted something I'd clearly overlooked a hundred times. Tucked into the clear front pocket was a small booklet titled: *The PHARMSI CHECK: A Checking System to Prevent Dispensing Errors* (see *Toolkit*).

It was a lifeline. I absorbed every word as if it were Scripture. The next day, I marched into work, scribbled *PHARMSI* in all caps on a dispensing label, and stuck it to my station like a talisman. From then on, every time I dispensed a script, I worked the acronym through my mind as if it were oxygen until it became embedded in my memory. And here's the miracle: I got so good at checking, so precise in spotting potential harm, that the moment I fully registered, they handed me the honors of the checking bench. The reckless girl who couldn't get through a shift without ten near-misses was now guarding the gate.

And I am *grateful.* Grateful that my mistake didn't become a tragedy. Grateful that I was given the chance to repair what I almost shattered. Because sometimes, you need harsh wake-up calls to become the kind of pharmacist and person you are meant to be.

Unscript Yourself Echoes

#1: Mistakes aren't the enemy. Avoiding their meaning is. Guilt isn't the enemy either, but shame is.

Very few of us in pharmacy talk openly about the mistakes we've made. And yet, all of us have made them. That's because shame has made the topic radioactive. No one wants to be "that pharmacist,"—the one whose initials are in the near-miss column or the one who forgot to double-check. But here's what I've learned after standing in my own mistake and almost drowning in it: mistakes are not the enemy.

The real enemies are:

- Avoiding the meaning within the mistake.
- Shaming ourselves so deeply that we stop learning.
- Staying silent long enough that someone else makes the same error because we were too afraid to speak.

Here's the truth I wish were taught in pharmacy school and whispered at every staff meeting:

> Guilt says: "That action was wrong. How do I make it right?"
>
> Shame says: "I am wrong. How do I disappear?"

And far too often, we confuse the two. We wear shame like a uniform and call it "professional accountability." But it doesn't make us safer. It shrinks us. It makes us quiet. And in that silence, the system stays broken.

One of my favorite authors, Brené Brown, calls this out plainly: "Shame needs three things to grow exponentially: secrecy, silence, and judgment."[1]. And if that isn't a perfect summary of how pharmacy (and healthcare) systems treat error reporting, I don't know what is. We bury our mistakes in quality improvement folders and pretend we're better off for it. But secrecy doesn't build safety; it builds repetition.

The irony is that we have an entire field in healthcare called Clinical Quality Improvement. And yet we treat it like a backroom confessional instead of a learning space. We don't speak of it enough. And until we do, errors will keep happening, and healthcare systems will keep bleeding billions.

So here's the invitation: Don't fear your mistakes. Fear what happens when you pretend they don't exist.

#2: There's dignity in the thankless, but only if you name it.

Too often, we do work that goes unnoticed: packing blister packs, cleaning the CD safe, repeating ourselves to a confused patient for the fourth time, making lunches for toddlers, paying bills on time, and folding laundry that no one notices until it isn't done. We've all done that work, and when no one acknowledges it, it's tempting to believe it doesn't matter.

But when you don't name the meaning yourself, when you don't mentally, emotionally, or even spiritually affirm *why* that work matters, it doesn't just disappear. It erodes you. It becomes a form of silent suffering that quickly turns into resentment—a slow leak of purpose.

But if you name it, then you reclaim power. You reframe the struggle. You say:

- "This is building my patience."
- "This is sharpening my attention to detail."
- "This is forming the kind of leader I'd want to follow."
- "This is how I show love when I feel unseen."
- "This is my values in motion."

In both our professional and personal lives, many of us feel unseen. We do the hard, tedious, emotionally taxing jobs and feel erased by the system or by those closest to us. This is your permission to stop waiting for applause and to name the worth in what no one claps for. That is part of the Unscripting: refusing to let silence or invisibility define the meaning of your work.

#3: You don't need to love your job to take it seriously. You just need to know who pays the price when you don't.

It is far too easy to hunch under the weight of our burdens, to drown in the slow suffocation of mundaneness, to stew in resentment over a task we despise, replaying the same internal script that says, *This isn't why I studied. This isn't what I'm here for.*

But the dangerous part isn't the frustration. It's forgetting that on the other side of that mundane task—on the other end of that label, interaction, or repeat script refill—is a person. A human being whose fate, literally, may rest in our hands.

If there is one thing this experience taught me, it's that you do not need to love your job to honor it. You do not need to be inspired by the task to take it seriously. You only need to remember that when you don't show up fully present, entirely focused, and fully committed, someone else may pay the price.

I learned to detach my feelings from the function because feelings aren't always reliable. I trained myself to focus not on my mood, my job satisfaction, or how soul-dead the work felt that day, but on the sacredness of the responsibility—on the patient.

And this worked until something better arrived. Until I walked the path of purpose. Until I saw meaning in the work I once wanted to escape, and we'll uncover more of that transformation as this book unfolds. But for those who feel stuck in a role that doesn't align, let this serve as a simple, weighty awakening: treat every shift like your patient's life depends on it. Because it does.

Faith Echoes

Sometimes God's mercy doesn't look like rescue. It looks like a warning that came before the wreckage.

We don't always see it this way. When things fall apart, when error turns to consequence, when the diagnosis arrives, the mistake surfaces, or the dream disintegrates, it's far easier to blame God than to trust Him. It is far easier to accuse Him of absence than to search for His nearness, to question His wisdom rather than to ask what He is trying to reveal.

And Scripture doesn't ask us to shy away from that struggle because even the most devout cried out in confusion. Job—righteous, blameless, battered by loss—engaged in long, unfiltered dialogue with God. He didn't deny God's power, but he did question His justice. He demanded answers, challenged the silence, and wrestled with the divine weight that comes with asking, "Why me?" (Job 30–31).

I've asked those same questions many times, and I'm sure you have too. But here's what I've come to understand in hindsight: God's mercy doesn't always come packaged as a miracle. Sometimes it looks like the error that didn't escalate or the patient who caught what you missed. The moment that could have wrecked you but only bruised you instead.

In my case, the warning signs were everywhere—subtle promptings and intuitive nudges. The Holy Spirit whispers, *Slow down, realign, and pay attention.* But I refused to listen. I was too busy justifying my disconnection and too absorbed in my misery. So the lesson had to arrive in a form I couldn't ignore. And I'm grateful to God that when it did, it didn't destroy me.

That, I now believe, was an act of mercy.

Lamentations 3:22

"Because of the LORD's great love, we are not consumed, for his compassions never fail."

God was there—in the fact that the error wasn't severe enough to harm the patient, but was enough to wake me up, to help me realign and become a better pharmacist. And maybe that's what mercy looks like in its rawest form.

Unscript Yourself Toolkit

Permission to Forgive Yourself

One raw scribble beats a flawless essay.
No productivity guilt. This is a time for calibration.

Think of a mistake in your personal or professional life that still tugs at you. How has it shaped your character in the long run?

____

____

____

Name one task (at work or at home) that's breeding resentment. What meaning will you choose for it this week, without denying how you actually feel?

____

____

____

Where do you confuse guilt (repairable) with shame (identity-crushing) in your current season? Write one sentence that separates them.

____

____

____

Unscripted Permission Slips:

- You have permission to separate guilt from shame when things go sideways. Let guilt teach; send shame packing.
- You have permission to forgive your earlier self for not knowing what you know now.
- You have permission to find dignity in the thankless jobs, whether that's at home or work.

Unscripted Affirmation

I am not my mistakes. I name them, learn from them, and use them as a tool for growth.

Unscripted Tips

For the complete PHARMSI check guide, visit:
https://www.pda.org.nz/
open the *Resources* tab, and scroll down to **The PHARMSI Check** at the bottom of the page.

PHARMSI is not a magic bullet to eliminate errors; but, for many pharmacists, it is a powerful tool to improve efficiency and reduce risk. It was developed after thorough literature reviews, pharmacist surveys, reference to human factors psychology and ergonomics, pilot testing and user feedback. Despite all this, it is relatively simple!

PHARMSI was developed through four steps:

1. **Determining the essential parts of the final check** and ranking them in order of importance.
2. **Reversing the check order** so the least important parts are checked first, and the most important parts are checked last. This "priority-recency" may help to maintain focus and attention.
3. **Linking check items** so that they follow one another in a logical order.
4. **Streamlining the check**, using the prescription label as a guide (when viewed in a simple clockwise pattern).

The name **PHARMSI** itself is the *mnemonic code* for the final safety check.

P	=	**Patient**
H	=	**How to take = Directions**
A	=	**Amount total = Quantity**
R	=	**Route = Form**
M	=	**Medicine Name = Drug**
S	=	**Strength**
I	=	**Interactions *(and other notes)***

CHAPTER 5

You Are Forged in the Fire

That which does not kill us makes us stronger.

—Friedrich Nietzsche

One of the most important lessons I carried forward from my internship year, particularly after that dispensing error, is that preparing prescriptions isn't only about excellent service or getting the patient out the door with a smile. It is a negotiation between two competing priorities: efficiency and accuracy. Lean too far toward speed, and you risk safety in the name of service. Tip too far toward perfectionism, and you drive yourself and your team to the brink of burnout.

I've lived at both edges—rushing on bad days and overchecking on worse ones. I learned that it's about providing calibrated care. For a newbie pharmacist, it takes time to find that safe balance, and it takes even longer to practice maintaining it. But it's that hard-earned and often imperfect balance that makes you not just any pharmacist, but one with a reputation that precedes you.

During that year, I saw the profound impact pharmacists have on saving lives. One afternoon, a man walked in, pale and sweating, shivering violently. He was slurring slightly, hunched over the counter, muttering that he just needed some lozenges for his sore throat. "The doctor said they don't have any appointments today," he said, trying to wave me off with that dismissal people use when they're trying not to fall apart.

With my pharmacist's gut instinct—those moments when you sense something is off, and the red flags fire in your brain—I empathetically said, "I know you feel unwell. I'm not selling you anything because you should see a doctor. I'll call them for you."

I was tasked with weekly visits to drop off medical supplies at the local medical center, which immensely helped me build a working relationship with local medical providers. I've always seen this adversarial tension with some doctors, but I was forced early on to learn how to shape that dynamic. I learned that if you don't walk into a new clinic, introduce yourself, and make a good impression, you can't exactly complain when the doctor bristles at your suggestion to halve the dose.

That relationship helped me pick up the phone without hesitation, give the nurse a rundown of this patient's symptoms, and ask if she could squeeze him in, which she did within the hour. A few hours later, the nurse called me back and said, "Thank you for referring him. He had sepsis secondary to untreated strep throat. We've started him on IV antibiotics."

I had saved my first life. My preceptor was proud, which said something given the gazillion errors he'd caught in those first few months. And part of me—quietly and sheepishly—hoped this minor act of clinical conviction might make up for all my past transgressions. The script had shifted.

As strenuous as that year was, my preceptor nurtured in me the discipline of looking beyond the paper. Knowledge of holistic health and root-cause thinking that didn't come through lectures. It came through watching how he asked better questions. How he treated the prescription not as the solution but as the start of the investigation. What else is going on in that patient's life that is contributing to the condition they've presented with?

It's easy to fall into the grind of checking prescriptions and pushing them out the door, staying laser-focused on the label, the MIMS note, and the interaction flag. I've been guilty of that too—of letting the system's urgency hijack my intention. But when I paused for an extra moment and looked beyond the script long enough to be curious, I started asking:

- Why are they on so many medications?
- Is this a prescribing cascade?
- Are they taking a medicine to counter the side effects of another medicine?
- Are they tolerating symptoms they think are "just part of life," when, in fact, they are pharmacological side effects no one ever explained?

How many elderly patients do we see who walk around with chronic fatigue, dry mouth, incontinence, and indigestion, wearing these symptoms like a badge of old age? But we know that too often it's not just age. It's amlodipine, or oxybutynin, or sertraline, or the fifth medication in a list someone stopped reviewing years ago. And therein lies one of a pharmacist's hidden superpowers. It's in that candid conversation over the counter—the single question that shifts someone from passive recipient to informed participant in their own care.

This is why I repeat: Pharmacists will not be replaced by AI. Not the ones who pause, who ask, who connect with the patient beyond the script with empathy and understanding. Algorithms don't see a frail man trying to mask his dizziness, and they certainly don't say, "You don't look well. I'll call the clinic for you." We save lives not only by catching errors but by seeing what everyone else missed. And we do that best when we look beyond the script and into the patient's story.

We save lives not only by catching errors but by seeing what everyone else missed.

I also believe we've created a world where there's a pill for every ill, a system that reflexively medicates before it ever investigates. We've built healthcare like an ambulance at the bottom of the cliff, but we rarely focus on building fences at the top. Without detouring too far into the politics of prevention, this is also why I think pharmacists sit at the intersection of clinical intervention and community connection. In that space lies a radical opportunity not just to dispense, but to educate, to guide, and to point upstream and ask, "What would happen if we caught this earlier?"

I share this because these perspectives didn't just shift how I practiced; they became the root of my career—the skills I nurtured, leaned into, and was hired for. They became my language, the lens through which I speak in all my board discussions, and the lane in which I operate. In time, they became one of the clearest ways I could offer value to patients beyond what the system provides—value beyond the title.

If you have years in your career that you have a love-hate relationship with, I can totally relate. These are the years that broke you yet shaped you. There were so many moments when academic pressure met emotional exhaustion in a head-on collision, and I found myself calling the intern support team yet again, sobbing. The trigger was almost always buried assignments. My preceptor, bless him, had this maddening habit of letting my completed assignments sit on his desk, where they would slowly sink beneath piles of paper. So I developed what essentially became my year-long mantra: "I'm so sorry. It's done. But he hasn't signed it off yet." I said it so many times that the intern coordinator would pick up the phone and immediately say, "It's okay. I know, I know."

And don't get me started on my calculations test. To reach the final registration exam, every trainee must pass a nerve-dismantling calculations test—the kind that's designed to assess your dose accuracy under what they lovingly call "normal pharmacy conditions." You know, phones ringing nonstop, a baby screaming three aisles away, someone asking where the iron tablets are while another demands to speak to the pharmacist about why their metoprolol looks different. The norm that only you will understand.

Well, I failed that test. Not once, but twice! Failing a third time meant no entry to the final pre-registration exam. So no registration, no qualification. And the entire year? Flushed. It wasn't because I couldn't do math. In every role since, I've been *the* go-to person for double-checking calculations—IV infusions, palliative conversions, you name it—went through me. But by the end of that year, I was fried from the inside out.

Sometimes it's like driving with the fuel light glaring; workplace pressures crush your spirit until there's only enough in reserve to reach the next petrol station. Layer on the emotionally taxing assignments, the ever-present threat of error, the bureaucratic chaos of an internship (and, for me, the first year of marriage), and suddenly it's a pressure cooker. There is no breathing space or recovery, just that constant undertone whispering, *Don't screw this up.*

I sat the test for the third time, and somehow my preceptor, intentionally or not, made it even more nerve-wracking than it already was, as if the concept of normal pharmacy conditions weren't already ridiculous enough in a testing environment. I completed it, but then there was the agony of waiting for him to mark it. As per usual, he took it, placed it in its sacred spot on his desk (that haphazard pile), and there it sat for a few days.

There is nothing worse than knowing your fate lies in someone else's hands, so I waited along with the internship supervisor, pulling not just my hair out, but my fate too. Eventually, he marked it, and by grace, I passed. Barely!

The final scrutiny came right before I got signed off for my pre-registration exam. And, of course, it had to involve the one thing I thought I was halfway decent at: compounding. Despite my best efforts, I became the poster child for specks in creams and ointments—"invisible-to-the-human-eye" specks. Specks I was blind to, but that my preceptor could spot from across the dispensary with supernatural precision.

I had just finished a cream mixture, polished it, scraped it, and he, calm as ever, leaned in, took one look, and announced, "There's a speck." I stared at him, then squinted back at the cream, turned it under the light, but saw nothing. According to him, it didn't pass the standard. And with that, he calmly informed me he would not sign me off to attend the registration exam because my compounding did not meet the required standard.

After a year of errors, overdue assignments, spiritual exhaustion, and clawing my way back to clinical competence, I honestly felt like I couldn't take one more knock. I felt devastated, not because of the cream, but because of what the cream represented: that after everything, I still wasn't enough. These are moments when your body stills, as if it has just received the final blow, when you don't have it in you to cry or argue. I stared at the cream, then grabbed my spatula again and scraped the living hell out of it, like it was the only thing between me and my destiny. If the slab could feel, it would have cried out from the sheer force I applied to it. Eventually, after what felt like hours, he sighed, nodded, and said, "All right. That'll do."

He mercifully signed me off for the pre-registration exam. Another mountain, but at least this time I could see the summit. I packed my bag with more anxiety than clothing and traveled for the exam. The experience wasn't nearly as terrifying as I had expected because, in the real world, you're not only dealing with one case at a time under timed pressure; you're calculating creatinine clearance while a child is screaming bloody murder across the counter. You're deciphering the doctor's handwriting from two days ago while being asked where the cough syrup is and navigating a substitution call from the doctor's office. You're managing real people, with real chaos and real emotions. And that's what makes pharmacists so brilliant. It's not the textbooks or passing the exams. It's the ability to function clinically and compassionately in absolute madness. All sarcasm aside, there's something sacred about that!

If you've ever arrived at an end goal or a destination too tired to appreciate the fruit of your labor, then you'll know what I mean when I say I passed. Finally. No fanfare. Just a quiet exhale and the slow realization that maybe I had earned this.

You'll have had hardships in your career—many of them. Setbacks that felt personal. Delays, tears, humiliations. But those very moments, the ones you hated at the time, the ones that made you want to quit, are the same ones that shape you into the pharmacist you are today.

As much as I would've liked an easier version of events, I wouldn't want my journey to have gone any differently, because it forged something in me I didn't know I needed. People often ask me in podcast interviews, in that casual, throwaway manner, "If you could go back, what would you do differently?" The answer they expect is some shiny-sounding lesson. But my answer is always the same: *Nothing.* If I had done one thing differently, I wouldn't have landed exactly here, a place where I'm glad to be, because *here* means I made it. I can't justify rewriting anything about the past if it means forfeiting this version of the present.

No experience goes to waste—even the parts you want to erase and the parts that almost break you. There is a lesson buried inside every day if you're willing to pay attention. And those who learn to notice are the ones who outlast, outgrow, and outshine the trajectory the system has set for them. That year was a crucible in every sense of the word (emotionally, spiritually, professionally), and there were more days I cried than I didn't. But I am grateful to my preceptor for not giving up on me and for pushing me despite feeling the unfairness. Without the pressure, I wouldn't be the pharmacist I am today.

I chose to let that year make me rather than break me. I've made peace with it and embraced it with all its chaos and contradictions, its small wins and emotional collapses, because the hardest things you will walk through are often the ones that gift you the most. As I've grown in my career and life, I've stopped wishing for ease and started recognizing the gifts found in hard seasons. They rip open old scaffolding and invite something stronger to take root. Resilience doesn't come from winning; it comes from withstanding the challenges, embracing growth despite the chaos, and choosing resilience amidst the tears that you don't always dare to let fall.

Resilience doesn't come from winning; it comes from withstanding the challenges, embracing growth despite the chaos, and choosing resilience amidst the tears that you don't always dare to let fall.

After the long hours, the tests, the tears, and the slow forging of confidence, I walked into a season of the aspirational young pharmacist—one who has found her footing but not yet her place. One who wants to make her mark, advocate for change, and do more than just follow orders, but discovers that the tide against her is far stronger than anything she endured as an intern.

It's a season I know too many of you have faced and perhaps still do—one that rarely gets spoken about but is carried quietly and courageously behind the scenes.

Unscript Yourself Echoes

#1: You're not "Just a Pharmacist."

Have you ever whispered that quieter lie to yourself at some point: "I'm just a pharmacist." If you are reading this while barely holding it together, doubting your worth because your white coat doesn't come with a hospital badge or prescribing rights, then I need you to stop and rethink that narrative.

That story is the quiet erosion of self-worth that I was trapped in for years. It's not yours. It was handed to you by a healthcare system that has undervalued pharmacists for decades. That expected you to be both the safety net and the scapegoat.

And when those narratives get replayed—verbally and internally—they do more than bruise your confidence. They fracture your vision. They blur the long-term view of what this profession could be. And slowly, insidiously, they chip away at your sense of purpose. It's not the hours or the exhaustion that deplete you. It's the quiet, unspoken belief that says you don't matter. But the reality is that you don't just catch errors or correct doses. You are the connector, the empathetic communicator, the one who often catches what others miss, and that's when you save lives.

#2: Healing isn't always found in what we prescribe. It's often hidden in what we overlook.

When I graduated from pharmacy school, I believed that healing was found in medicines, that intervention equals action, and that treatment means ticking a box and moving on. But as I progressed in my career, I learned that healing is not only found in medicines. It hides in the question, "*Are you sleeping?*" In noticing that a patient has been in three times this week with a foggy look and a fading appetite. In realizing that side effects don't just show up on MIMS, they show up in someone's life who is now standing before you.

We weren't taught to bill for these moments. We weren't always shown how to track them in a workflow system. But this is where healing begins: in the pause and the human connection. Because healing isn't just a script; it's a redirection toward what still hurts the patient but hasn't yet been named. It lies in what the system overlooks.

I've learned that becoming an indispensable pharmacist comes from taking time to know your patients, building rapport at the counter, being empathetic, and connecting with the human beyond the script.

Faith Echoes

You are not meant to survive your calling alone.

I wish I could tell you I handled that year with grace, that I prayed harder, journaled more, or found some grounding ritual that carried me through. But I was just trying to survive. My body was brittle from the lack of sleep, and the adrenaline surges that came with every "you've failed" that echoed after a horrifying mistake.

My faith flickered not because I stopped believing, but because I didn't have the emotional bandwidth to wrestle with God the way I usually would. I felt spiritually frayed, relationally thin, and mentally stretched. Even my marriage—this brand-new, still-fresh union—became a background casualty to the pressure. I was disappearing into this endless swirl of proving myself and not being enough.

That year not only tested my clinical knowledge; it tested my nervous system, my ability to cope, and my faith. And it taught me what no textbook ever will: You don't have to burn out to be in danger. Sometimes you quietly hollow out. And if you're not careful, if you don't pause long enough to notice, you might not realize you're empty until there's nothing left to pour from.

You've got to catch yourself before you disappear into the doing, into the unraveling and the stress, by remembering God through it all. God never asks you to survive your calling alone. He invites you to walk with Him through it. Even when you can't feel His presence, and when you forget how to pray, He will always be there: quiet, steady, and holding what you can no longer hold. He wants you broken and messy because that's when His strength is magnified.

Psalm 73:26:

My flesh and my heart may fail, but God is the strength of my heart and my portion forever.

Unscript Yourself Toolkit

Permission to Let the Hard Make You, Not Break You

Light a candle or take a walk. No need for productivity guilt. This is calibration. One true line per prompt is better than ten perfect ones.

Can you think of a particular person or manager who, though tough on you at the time, ultimately sharpened you? What was the lesson? What habit did it forge in you?

What would help you thrive in your current role that you haven't yet shared with your supervisor? What would make it safer or easier to share it?

When you feel pressured or scrutinized at work, do you speak up? Why or why not?

Unscripted Permission Slips

- You have permission to practice calibrated care, not perform perfection.
- You have permission to be the one who builds the fence at the top of the cliff—the one who keeps patients from falling in the first place.
- You have permission to stop fighting the hard times that shaped you, accept them for what they were, grieve what they cost you, and carry forward the wisdom without dragging the weight.

Unscripted Affirmation

I am a pharmacist forged in the fire, not defined by it.
I practice calibrated care, ask brave questions, and bring my whole human self into every decision I make.

PART III

The Conflict

Not everybody can be famous,
but everybody can be great because
greatness is determined by service.

—MARTIN LUTHER KING JR.

CHAPTER 6

Your Worth Is Not Measured by Their Insecurities

You are not intimidating. They are intimidated by your attitude and success. Big difference.

—Unknown

I bid farewell to my internship, joined the ranks of pharmacists, and braced for the joy of the checking bench. It happened a few days before Christmas because that's when chaos in community pharmacy usually hits. While the only other staff member was on lunch and I was running the dispensary solo—dispensing, checking my work, and trying to hold the fort—a patient came to collect their script. One I had self-checked but not yet bagged. Just as I went to hand it over, something made me pause. I glanced down, and my gut flipped. I had labeled the box "fluoxetine" instead of "tramadol," not because the names were similar, but because the generic packaging was identical. I made a quiet U-turn and slipped back into the dispensary, my heart pounding so hard I could feel it in my ears. I paused and took a deep breath. Somewhere between the third inhale and the fourth exhale, I knew: *I cannot keep doing this.*

I had caught the error. But what if I hadn't? What if next time I'm too tired, too stretched, too distracted trying to survive the day solo that I don't? I never want to be in a place where my stress becomes a risk to someone else's body—not again!

Leaving that workplace was one of the hardest decisions I've ever made because, despite the pressures, I felt tethered to my preceptor, who had poured time and tough love into me. I was raised to believe you don't walk out on people who invest in you. But I was wrecked from working alone, and I felt like I needed a fresh start—the kind that didn't smell like last week's leftover scripts and half-swallowed resentment.

There are times in your career when you don't justify the dollars you're receiving for the amount of work you're putting in. I was paid only a few dollars more than an intern, despite being a fully qualified pharmacist, and was often left to work solo. I had no second check and no team to lean on. It was just me and the mounting pressure that made my jaw ache and my shoulders curl in on themselves. It was about knowing my worth, and I hadn't yet found mine.

As I moved forward in my career, chasing stability and some form of recognition, I realized that money isn't everything. It sounds obvious when said out loud, but when you're desperate to feel seen, to be compensated in a way that matches your exhaustion, you don't always listen to obvious truths.

I've seen too many pharmacists make the same mistake I did, jumping for the dollars without checking the ground they were landing on. Sometimes that bigger paycheck is wrapped in barbed wire. The shifts are longer, the politics are thicker, the staff are territorial, and every unresolved issue gets handed to the newbie as some warped form of initiation. I learned the hard way that a place that pays you less but supports you more is worth more than a place that throws money at you to keep you behind the counter and cut off from patients, from learning, from purpose itself. Pay can cover bills, yes, but it cannot quiet the ache of being stuck.

I resigned and moved on to the very employer who had once promised me an internship, only to withdraw it when the winds of management changed—the same one I had worked at during my summer breaks. So when they offered me a role now, I told myself it made sense.

I already knew the system, and it felt safe and familiar.

I should have known better. Not because they'd burned me once, though they had, but because everything in my gut was whispering, *Don't go back just because you know the way.* But I was tired and grateful for an offer. Deep down, I still wanted to prove something—to them, to myself, to the version of me who once begged them for a spot. I followed my ego over my brain. I wanted to show them they were wrong to reject me the first time. Little did I know I wasn't returning to a workplace; I was returning to a wound, hoping maybe this time it would heal differently. Turns out, God knew better.

Growing up as a migrant in New Zealand, I watched my parents build businesses, armed with nothing but grit, broken English, and faith that made no logical sense. They embodied hard work and resilience in the face of every closed door. They carved those traits in me, and I absorbed them like gospel. What I didn't realize—what I'm still learning, painfully and slowly—is that this high-performing, strive-for-better rhythm I inherited doesn't always land well with people. I hate how arrogant that sounds, but the truth I've learned the hard way is that intensity makes people uncomfortable. What feels like growth to you can feel like competition to the insecure. And what feels like honoring my family's legacy can, apparently, come off as threatening. And that came back to bite me. Hard.

At that pharmacy, there was one pharmacist who harassed and bullied me until I broke. After the year I had just survived, this felt like execution in a public arena. For starters, I was an early-career pharmacist, the unspoken job title for *resident pharmacy slave.* They gave me the jobs nobody else wanted, as if the entire workflow hierarchy had flipped and I didn't get the memo. It felt like déjà vu from last year. Think Cinderella, but instead of the Godmother, outright bullying by Hades from the Underworld, showing up every day in scrubs and passive aggression, with mocking, name-calling, and jokes that were like verbal shrapnel wrapped in fake laughter. The stuff that leaves no physical mark but bruises your sense of self until you stop trusting your own instincts. At some point in your career, you likely faced it too. Bullying in pharmacy is rampant. It hides behind titles, behind tired excuses like "That's just how she is," or "He means nothing by it." But it's there. And

I wish that I had known my rights; that someone had handed me a copy of the employment law handbook before I ever touched a MIMS. I wish someone had taught us at university how to draw workplace boundaries with the same confidence that we were taught to counsel on clopidogrel.

I remember one particular scenario (classic corporate pharmacy theatrics) where management imposed sales targets, KPIs, the whole shiny spreadsheet of "performance metrics." I didn't push for numbers; I just spoke like a human and never missed my targets. Management was thrilled and applauded my results. But the other pharmacists? Well, not so much. The tension became thick and passive when they accused me of being "too forward" and "too ambitious," as if those were crimes. Eventually, I was banned from the shop floor, which was the one part of the job I actually loved—talking to patients. I was told to stick to the back, focus on "dispensary duties," and leave the front of house to someone else. So I was back behind the bench with my eyes off patients, my voice muted, and my spirit shrinking.

Perhaps the only true highlight of that entire year was the time I caught a shoplifter on a quiet Saturday evening. I was half-dreaming in the dispensary, head propped up, trying to survive the last hour of the shift, when I glanced out at the shop floor and saw her slipping a perfume bottle into her son's bag. Not her bag, but his, so he wouldn't be flagged as underage. And there I was, shooting out from behind the dispensary like some overworked retail avenger. It so happened that, in the middle of the chaos, an undercover police officer was walking past and jumped in. Perfect timing. A sting operation without the planning. Who knew I had an eye for catching thieves? I couldn't stop workplace sabotage, but at least I could stop a stolen Chanel No. 5.

And just when I thought I had adjusted to the slow burn of daily disrespect, the pharmacy gods delivered one final blow—the kind you don't bounce back from. It all came to a head when I was falsely accused of a dispensing error—one I didn't commit. My signature had allegedly been on a script I had never laid eyes on. The setup was immaculate, and I looked guilty. I even felt guilty, though I couldn't recall a thing about the incident. I crumbled under the weight of it all. It wasn't until legal support pushed for a camera review that the footage proved I wasn't present when the error occurred. And did anyone face any consequences for forging my signature, accusing me of an error I didn't make, and nearly collapsing my career in its infancy? You bet not. Not a warning or a conversation. Just silence, as if the entire ordeal had never happened.

It was a far more emotionally taxing year than the one before it because I was already running on a deficit. The system seemed determined to keep overdrawing from my account, from my energy, from my trust, and from my fragile belief that pharmacy could still be a place of care.

Some seasons don't only exhaust you; they hollow you, siphoning out joy until all that's left is anger braided with resentment. You replay moments in your head, wishing you had spoken or stood up for yourself because it feels as though something sacred was stolen from you—the right to a workplace that was safe, the right to colleagues who didn't weaponize power, the right to a profession that didn't demand daily survival tactics. And yet, the bitter irony is that the resilience we now carry, the character that can stand in the fire without disintegrating, was forged in those very silences we once endured.

The resilience we now carry, the character that can stand in the fire without disintegrating, was forged in those very silences we once endured.

You won't be surprised to learn that I resigned twelve months later. One full rotation around the sun and one full year of proving to myself that just because you can endure something doesn't mean you should. Your worth is not diminished by the choice to quit; if anything, it is revealed in the dignity to walk away.

Once again, I found myself in the vicious cycle of job applications, each more disheartening than the last. It didn't look good to leave two roles in a row. It made me look unstable and feel even more so. It didn't matter how valid the reasons were because, on paper, I came across as a red flag. I applied for over thirty roles, and after more than fifteen interviews, I landed a junior community pharmacist job.

You may wonder why I kept getting rejected despite my experience. And I wish I had a more flattering answer. But the truth is, I had no references from previous roles because I left even though they wanted me to stay. And secondly? I was terrible at interviews. They spun my nerves into tangled knots and stripped every ounce of confidence from me. I was a terrible speaker, which may come as a surprise given how prolific I am now in writing and speaking. The only way to get better at anything is to keep failing at it until it stops scaring you. After what felt like my hundredth interview, I can assure you I was no longer fazed. Not because I had grown confident, but because I had become comfortably numb.

And amidst all that chaos, rejection, and growing numbness, the universe threw me a seismic jolt: I fell pregnant—something I neither planned nor anticipated. I feel guilty saying it, but I felt crushed. This wasn't news I welcomed when I was still trying to find my footing in a profession that already felt like it was crushing me sideways. Nor was it something I wanted to come up in the middle of a job application, just as I was trying to prove I was reliable, responsible, and career-ready. I kept thinking, *They're going to think I'm not dependable, that I don't have my life in order, that I don't plan things properly.*

Despite the shame, I blamed God. I remember whispering into my pillow, *Why would You let this happen now?* I wasn't being ungrateful. I know children are a gift; I just wasn't whole enough to receive that gift. I was too bruised, too exhausted, too uncertain about everything, and I was still trying to patch together my own identity, let alone become responsible for someone else's.

I didn't know who or how to ask for advice on what to do next. *Do I say something now? Do I disclose it in the interview? Do I deserve to be applying right now?* Surviving without that income, with a baby on the way, was not achievable. This wasn't something I could list on my CV: *P.S. I'm pregnant and will require maternity leave in T-minus nine months. Please hire me anyway?*

So I did the only pragmatic thing I could think of: I applied as if nothing had changed. I didn't add it to the CV or mention it in cover letters. I just hoped they'd meet me, see my potential, and that maybe, by the time I told them, they'd be too committed to turn away. That they'd support me through the process and be ready to welcome me back after maternity leave. It felt wrong and manipulative, yet it also felt necessary. Because even in my uncertainty, I was still worthy of opportunity, worthy of joy, but I felt unsafe talking about it. Eventually, someone saw the potential behind the brokenness, and I was hired.

But once again, I'll blame the system that makes it so hard for women in the workforce to be whole humans. Why did this have to be such a hard conversation to have? Why isn't it normalized in society, even more so in our profession? If we, health professionals, can't muster the empathy and understanding needed for a situation like this, then how on earth can we expect society to do better?

To say I was morally collapsing is an understatement. I felt incompetent and hollow on the inside. At that point, I was running on autopilot with a lot of I-hate-Monday energy, showing up in the last few weeks of my current role because I had to, smiling because it was expected. And that's not exactly the mindset you want to carry into a new job, but it was all I had left after two years of unrelenting moral injury.

Shame of pregnancy, bullying, and forged accusations tried to destroy my self-worth. But worth is not borrowed, forged, or stolen; it is God-given and remains intact, no matter what rooms or people try to rewrite it. Your worth is not measured by someone else's insecurities or by the circumstances; it is measured by your response. And when that response is anchored in dignity, faith, and values, you have already won the test of life. These wounds don't erase your purpose; instead, they redirect you toward it.

Unscript Yourself Echoes

#1: Obligation is not a calling.

Sometimes the hardest thing to walk away from isn't the role; it's the version of yourself that believed staying was the noble thing to do. But staying small to keep others comfortable is not loyalty, because loyalty that costs your health or risks another life isn't loyalty; it's self-betrayal.

Burnout isn't a badge; it's a warning sign. When the systems we work in become louder than the voice inside us and wear us down, mistakes are inevitable. Listening to your stress isn't a weakness; it's wisdom. If you're at a point where you're working from obligation and burnout, it's okay to pause and rethink whether your work aligns with the version of you that serves your highest calling or whether you are depleting your soul.

#2: More money doesn't mean more meaning.

I know you hear that statement all the time, usually from people who already have plenty of it. But let me tell you why they say it: Once you've reached a place of financial comfort, it becomes blindingly clear that more money won't fix the ache inside you. I've been there. I chased the rise. I hit the income goal. And I still found myself asking, "*Is this it?*"

Research indicates that after your basic needs, comforts, and a little extra are met, the connection between money and happiness plateaus. What actually nourishes you will need to come from within. From looking inward. From inner alignment.

Some positions will throw money at you while stripping your autonomy, suffocating you with KPIs, letting colleagues mistreat you, and demanding your weekends in exchange for soul erosion. So, a job that pays slightly less but grants you breathing space, support, freedom, and room to grow is worth more than another $10,000 you can't enjoy because you're too depleted to live. If the paycheck is padded but your soul is shrinking, it's not a promotion; it's a trap. Some jobs pay you in dollars, but the right ones pay you in dignity.

#3: Your light will always expose someone else's shadows.

When you grow, when you become so good at something that you begin to shine, it doesn't only inspire; it disrupts. It unsettles people who aren't ready to confront their own stagnation. But they won't say that.

Oprah Winfrey said it best: "You are built not to shrink down to less but to blossom into more."[1] So, if your growth is causing discomfort to those around you, let it be confirmation that you're getting

Unscripted—that your becoming is expanding beyond the script they had for you. Their reaction is never your responsibility, and their values are not your truth, so let their discomfort be data that you are stepping into your destiny.

Faith Echoes

#1: Why is God patient with those who hurt us?

When things go against us and injustice takes its toll, we expect God to swoop in and punish the wrongdoer, restore what was lost, and declare our innocence. That's the justice we crave: quick, clean, and immediate. But that's not how God works.

When you've been hurt and the lies told about you roar louder than the truth ever could. When the people who harmed you walk freely while you collapse under the weight of false accusations and betrayal. And when it feels like the world is conspiring and everyone is turning their back, these are the faith-testing times.

I've learned that God's vengeance doesn't arrive like courtroom justice. He doesn't swoop in with a lightning bolt. He is kind, patient, and a God of second chances. Because the people who hurt you are His children too, sometimes He waits not to punish them, but to give them one more chance to repent, to bring the truth forward, and to choose light. And if they don't? We have to believe God is never mocked, that heaven keeps better records than HR ever will.

If you never live to see your reputation restored, know this:

Romans 12:19 (ESV): "*Vengeance is mine, I will repay, says the Lord.*"

Perhaps you'll never live to see your rights earned back on Earth, but you've got to trust in God's wisdom and fairness. He may well allow them to get away with it, but God won't forget what happened. Because when no one else advocates for you, heaven still holds a record, and your name will not be erased.

#2: God wants you real and raw.

Have you ever wanted something so badly, but when you finally get it, you're not grateful for it? You can believe in miracles and still not be ready for them. You can know a child is a blessing and still feel broken by the weight of their arrival. You can trust God and still yell at Him through a clenched jaw when His timing bulldozes your plans.

I used to hold on to this ideal image of the "good believer" who was always grateful, always blissful, and always doing the right thing. I strived to be that believer, but I struggled when I didn't conform. As I delved into the book of Psalms, I realized that that is not the relationship God wants. God doesn't want sugar-coated sanctity. He wants you raw, real, and unfiltered. He wants you with your messiness, ingratitude, and doubts, like David. He wants you broken so He can heal you, humble so He can lift you, and doubtful so that you can find rest in Him.

I've learned that God doesn't want us to fake gratitude or hide our weaknesses and insecurities. He wants us to voice our anger to Him and talk through our insecurities because He is the real Father in heaven who wants to share the load. He doesn't want polished perfection. He wants truth and submission. Raw honesty is not disloyalty to your faith; it's the first language of healing.

Davidic Honesty: Psalm 142:2

"I pour out before him my complaint; before him I tell my trouble."

Unscript Yourself Toolkit

Permission to Walk Away to Protect Your Peace

Go through this with your whole heart.
One line of truth can light more than a hundred rehearsed ones.

Can you recall a time when every part of you whispered it was time to walk away, yet you stayed? Or perhaps you finally left. What story did you tell yourself in that moment, and what did it cost or save you?

___

___

___

Think back to a moment when someone's words or actions bruised you in the workplace. How did you respond? With silence, confrontation, or escape? How did that choice shape the way you see yourself now?

___

___

___

If you had to safely disclose a painful truth today (about pregnancy, burn-out, bullying, etc.), who could you trust with it? What would you need to feel protected when speaking it aloud?

___

___

___

Unscripted Permission Slips

- You have permission to treat a near-miss not as proof you're careless, but as a holy wake-up call that your soul is asking for change.
- You have permission to stop chasing pay raises that come wrapped in barbed wire. Your true currency is dignity, growth, and the space to breathe.
- You have permission to stop letting your worth be weighed on the shaky scales of someone else's insecurities.

Unscripted Affirmation

My worth is not in the job, the title, the paycheck, the manager's mood, or the rumor mill. My worth is inherent, and I carry it in how I've endured, in how I've come this far, and in the faith and values I choose to live by.

Unscripted Tips: What I Wish I Knew

#1: How to Deal with Bullying

- Keep a dated log (who, what, where; verbatim phrases; witnesses).
- Document everything, even small comments or microaggressions. They form a pattern.
- Seek legal or union support early, before you're in crisis. You deserve safety, not just survival.
- Save emails and screenshots, and follow up on verbal incidents via email.
- Ask for a support person in meetings.
- Know the escalation ladder (manager → HR → external body/union).
- Know your rights and familiarize yourself with your local employment regulations and helplines. Don't rely on managers to advocate for you. Be your own advocate.

#2: How to Assess a Job Opportunity

- Growth (mentorship, rotations, CPD)
- Autonomy (clinical time, initiatives)
- Safety (staffing ratios, second checks)
- Culture (bullying zero tolerance, escalation process)
- Flexibility (roster, breaks that actually happen)

CHAPTER 7

You Are Called to Purpose-Soaked Excellence

The will to win, the desire to succeed, the urge to reach your full potential . . . these are the keys that unlock the door to excellence.

—Confucius

I wasn't wired for compliance that made others comfortable, and I didn't push boundaries out of arrogance or question workflows just to be difficult. It was a slow-burning resistance born out of a deep, gnawing need to understand *why*. Why were we so bound to the phrase, "This is how it's always been"? Why did growth and innovation always seem to live on the other side of silence?

My manager didn't like that. He was a "head down, don't ask questions, get the job done" type. So he picked at me. It was a slow erosion that soaked me in self-doubt, offering backhanded praise wrapped in intense critique that it took me hours to realize I'd been insulted. He wanted compliance, and I brought curiosity. And that, it seemed, was the unforgivable sin. There were just enough quiet exclusions from meetings and discussions to make me wonder if I really was the problem.

► **PRO-TIP**

Curiosity gets mistaken for rebellion in systems that worship compliance. If you're the kind who asks why a little too often, don't shrink. You're not the problem. You're the pulse-check, and some will not like that, but keep being you.

To make matters worse, after returning from a six-month maternity leave, I was pregnant again. And I know what you're probably thinking: *Does she not believe in contraception?* Well, the crude pharmacist in me hated taking pills. Isn't it funny and darkly ironic how many pharmacists actually loathe medication? I chalk it up to the curse of knowledge. We know too much to be at peace with convenience. I shared the incredible news with my manager, who wasn't exactly congratulatory about it. It was like watching a CT scan light up across his face: "What the heck? You just got back from leave." Thankfully, the pharmacy owner was a woman who was gracious, empathetic, and quietly supportive. I think it was God's grace, plus my work ethic, that made the whole thing palatable enough to survive.

A few months rolled by, and I had my second daughter. But something inside me had shifted. When I returned from maternity leave the second time, I was done. Two years of shrinking, of being the problem just for being present, were enough. My absence from the workplace made the attitude toward me even more hostile. So I put in a formal complaint, not out of rage but with focused clarity. I told management exactly how the environment felt. I named the exclusion and the silencing. And for the first time, I felt empowered. To my manager's credit, he denied nothing.

We sat down for a formal meeting with management and HR. It was the first time I had ever been involved in an employment dispute, and I was terrified. I didn't know how to advocate for myself or what would happen afterward. *Would I be fired if I didn't prove myself? Will they believe me?* I was falling apart between words and sentences. So I prayed the lifeline prayer that somehow says everything: *God, I don't know how to do this. Please guide me.* And for two hours, we talked. It wasn't comfortable. There was a lot of "he did, she did" confrontation, but eventually, we reconciled. In the weeks that followed, things slowly got better.

For the first time in a long time, I was proud of having mustered the courage to stand up for myself, and I learned never to stay silent just because it's hard. Yes, the ground may shake, but the truth will give you inner stability.

Never stay silent just because it's hard.
Yes, the ground may shake,
but the truth will give you inner stability.

As time went by, I realized that what unsettled him wasn't my work ethic; it was my ability to catch mistakes, which he found confronting. I say that with no arrogance, only clarity. Because if he had seen me in my intern year, he would know the irony. He would know that that skill wasn't innate. It was born out of humiliation, of missteps, of a year spent learning the hard way what vigilance actually meant. I had learned the lesson so deeply that it rewired how I saw dispensing. I chased accuracy as if it were a matter of survival.

Eventually, my manager started to respect my way of practicing, so much so that one day he saw a call for members for the Pharmacy Council's Professional Conduct Committee—the panel that investigates pharmacist complaints—and offered to write a recommendation letter for me to apply for the appointment. I don't think he realized he was doing me the biggest favor of my career. I remember him shrugging and saying something like, "It's not a paid role, though." I thought, *Maybe that's why he isn't applying.*

But for me, the appointment itself mattered, even if I hadn't been paid, because the trust and recognition I would gain outweighed everything else. I thought, *Well, I doubt I'd get it anyway, what with my record-breaking error history and barely three years of practice under my belt.* But I had the letter of recommendation, so I gave it a shot in the dark. I figured, at best, they'd recognize my name next time I apply, and, at worst, it would remind me how far I still have to go.

And this time I didn't have to shrink to be chosen. I got the appointment. And it was paid! That's when I realized that excellence didn't need to be my defense mechanism anymore; it was becoming my doorway into the Call to More—the kind of Unscripted purpose that takes root when you refuse to shrink, even if that comes at a cost. And

► PRO-TIP

The biggest career lesson I've learned is to delay the money chase. I'm not promoting working for free indefinitely, but there is immense value in doing something just to gain experience. Nearly everything I've built in my career, from writing to consulting, began by offering it for free in exchange for feedback and expertise. That currency compounds more than money.

just like that, without realizing it, I had taken my first steps on the Unscripted path.

This was how my career in governance began, and I often think about the irony of it all. If I hadn't been so catastrophically mistake-prone during my intern year—if I hadn't been mortified by how blind I was to the systems, the risks, the responsibilities—I might not have paid such obsessive attention to getting it right. Maybe I wouldn't have built the habit of slowing down when the pressure told me to speed up. Maybe I wouldn't have caught the errors that others missed. And I definitely wouldn't have arrived where I am today. Often, it's our biggest challenges that lead to life's most significant transformations. For that lesson, I'm eternally grateful to God.

Often, it's our biggest challenges that lead to life's most significant transformations.

One afternoon, a young man came in with a handwritten prescription for diazepam 5 mg and codeine 30 mg. This was not out of the ordinary, but something about it felt off. His energy was unsettled. I couldn't explain it, not in any way that would satisfy someone needing logic over intuition. I poked it under my manager's nose, who irritably waved it off: "It's fine. Just get on with it." But I couldn't let it go.

I remembered something my preceptor taught me—an odd little ritual that had seemed obsessive at the time: "If you ever doubt a prescription's authenticity, hold it up to the light. See if the ink shines through. Feel for the grooves of a real pen stroke." Authentic scripts (like people) leave an imprint.

And so I did. I turned it toward the light and tilted it in a few directions. I traced it with my fingertips, then checked the electronic dispensing history, and what I found chilled me. That same script had been dispensed in eight other pharmacies that week. I didn't panic. I simply walked outside. The man was sitting on a bench outside the pharmacy, posture hunched, looking extremely uncomfortable as I approached him. He had a "just hand over the drugs" look on his face.

"Is this for you, Mr. X?" I asked softly, letting the question linger in the air. Though I knew it was, I was trying to assess his response, perhaps to detect a shaky voice that would affirm my suspicions. "Yes, is there something wrong with it?" he replied, a tremble in his speech betraying a quiet dread. I didn't push. I simply asked if he had taken these medications before, to which he nodded discreetly. He appeared in terrible shape: pale, withdrawn in a way that screamed, *I'm not okay!*

I stepped back inside and called the police. My heart thudded the whole time, knowing that if I were wrong, I'd be punished for the chaos I was about to unleash and for falsely accusing someone of forgery. But if I were right, I might save a life. All the while, my manager stood off to the side, watching with a mix of irritation and cynical curiosity. It was hard to know whether he was amused by my so-called diligence or annoyed at what he clearly thought was wasted time.

The police came, and I led them to the young man. After they spoke to him for a while, the truth finally came out. He hadn't come to get high, nor to sell the drugs. He had come to die. He had been collecting enough codeine and diazepam from several pharmacies so that he could take his own life. And he was waiting on that bench, hoping I wouldn't notice. He left that day not with a bag of meds but with police officers, who gently took him to the psychiatric ward.

I'm sure you may have stories of catching script forgeries, too: patients presenting opioid prescriptions with that too-smooth confidence, the kind that evaporates the moment you say, "It'll be a ten-minute wait." And we step in to save their lives like detectives in disguise, despite our hearts pumping with fear of what may happen if they turn out to be connected to a gang or become threatening. By doing the right thing, we risk our safety; yet we still do it.

If I had kept my head down like a good junior pharmacist, followed orders, and trusted the script instead of my gut, that young man may well be dead. I think about that incident often, and it humbles me because that moment taught me something valuable: *Never ignore your inner voice.*

That incident became a hinge. The day I reported that gentleman's intent was the day I stepped into something I never thought I would: a responsibility that stretched beyond the dispensary into communities, cultures, and policies.

It was that incident that first brought me into contact with the police regarding drug misuse patterns in the communities. But it didn't stop there. The more I reflected on why that man, from a migrant background, felt suicide was his only option, the more I spoke out about cultural barriers, about the stigma surrounding mental health, and how invisible people become when they don't understand the systems they live within. Eventually, I was invited to meet the mayor of Christchurch, the city in which I lived. That conversation led to an unexpected appointment to chair the city's Multicultural Advisory Group—a group tasked with shaping how the local government could create safer, more inclusive environments, especially for migrants.

That appointment became the cornerstone of my work in Parliament three years later. But it all started in a pharmacy, on a quiet afternoon, because I listened to something deeper than protocol or another human.

None of this was a neat career plan. It was the Unscripted path unfolding. The vigilance in the dispensary led to governance at Council, which opened doors into community leadership and kept pointing me toward purpose. What felt like detours were actually directions. Some decisions won't come with protocols or policies. Some will ask you to choose between what's logical and what feels true. And when those moments come, you need to know where you stand. Trust the nudge, the sense that something is off when the paperwork says it isn't. That instinct is your moral compass. And when you do the right thing, the right thing eventually finds its way back to you.

When you do the right thing, the right thing eventually finds its way back to you.

One day, my manager sheepishly walked up to me with a furrowed brow and a tight jaw and said, "I'm worried the owner is going to demote me and put you in my place." I looked at him in quiet disbelief that my presence, my ideas (which were often ignored), and my work ethic could be seen as threatening. I didn't respond because I genuinely had no appropriate response. What do you say to someone who fears your growth more than they value your contribution?

I later came to understand that ideas die in theory more than in execution. They die when ego stands in the doorway, blocking the path for others. Think of how often your fresh ideas get buried under someone else's insecurity, and what could have been collaborative, expansive, future-shaping innovation gets dimmed out of fear it will outshine someone else. But dimming someone's brilliance will never make yours shine brighter; it makes the whole room darker. It's a frustrating reality that has impacted me throughout my career.

Ideas die in theory more than in execution. They die when ego stands in the doorway, blocking the path for others.

Once again, I found myself in silent self-negotiation: Maybe I should be a little less driven. A little less visible. A little less . . . good. I tried to suppress the urge to be excellent at what I do—to soften the edges of my competence, to ease back on the precision, to stop reaching so damn hard for better, to lean toward mediocrity. I tried to be less popular with patients, who kept returning and asking for me by name. To withhold a bit of the care I knew how to give so those around me wouldn't feel so exposed, so threatened. But I failed. For months, I lived in that space between knowing who I was and pretending not to be her—a state of spiritual whiplash.

Some days, I felt I had to "unbecome" the pharmacist I was meant to be just to keep the peace. It seemed that having a good work ethic was a threat, as if mediocrity were the price of acceptance. That broke something in me. The internal conflict grew louder, heavier, and palpable in a way I could feel in my whole body some days. I would stand at work and feel the whys orbiting: *Why should I shrink into mediocrity or follow a path that feels more like a cage than a calling?*

My life was carved through war, religious persecution, life-threatening events, and personal grief so grotesque I still don't know how I survived them. But they shaped me with wisdom, conviction, and an ability to defy all odds and always strive for better. I believe deep in my marrow that our truest calling is to serve and strengthen others with those wounds. That history, that pain, and that sharpening pushed me toward leadership and excellence—not perfection, but purpose-soaked excellence. The kind that says, "I will not waste what I've been through by playing small. I will lead by example and pass the ladder down for others to climb."

The truth is, there is a cost to this conviction. Excellence, especially in a system addicted to sameness, often makes people uncomfortable. It mirrors what they don't have. But that is the price of aligning with your purpose, with your highest self. That clarity in what you want is envied by those who don't know what they want from life. In the short term, it leads to growing pains. But in the long term, it leads you to your calling. So don't let the mediocrity of others and short-lived pain deprive you of long-term gains.

Unscript Yourself Echoes

#1: Pharmacists are detectives in disguise.

Pharmacists are the quiet gatekeepers. The guardians of medicines. The ones trained to check doses and drug interactions, as well as read the tension in someone's shoulders. To catch the tremble in a voice, and notice the details that don't quite add up. We are, whether or not anyone says it out loud, frontline harm reductionists in our communities.

We are also required to humbly use those skills even when the fast pace of the pharmacy tries to dull our senses. The pattern recognition, the discernment, the knowing without proof—these aren't skills taught at university, nor are they widely discussed in pharmacy. Rarely do pharmacists receive recognition for these innate skills. So the next time you catch that forged prescription, know that you are contributing not only to medication safety, but also to reducing harm and saving a life. Applaud yourself for that, because sometimes you need to be your own cheerleader to sustain the emotional side of the work you do.

#2: Being excellent isn't arrogance. It's obedience.

When I chose to traverse the Unscripted path—the one that doesn't conform, doesn't shrink, and doesn't wait for permission—I came across a quote by Oprah Winfrey that lodged itself so deeply into my bones it became liturgy: "Let excellence be your brand.... become so skilled, so vigilant, so flat-out fantastic that your talent cannot be dismissed." [1]

Those words became my mantra. Let them be yours too. You weren't made to be mediocre so others can feel comfortable. Your light will always be too bright for some rooms, but that's not a cue to dim it. That's a cue to illuminate. Because staying small isn't loyalty; it's a betrayal of the calling that lives inside you. You were meant and called for more, and if people and organizations keep dimming your light, you are in the wrong room. Don't let anyone shrink your excellence.

#3: Dimming someone's brilliance will never make your brilliance shine brighter. It only makes the room darker.

In the same vein, don't be the reason someone else's light flickers. Sometimes our actions—the words we don't say, the credit we withhold, the competitive mindset we justify as "professionalism"—can dim someone else's light.

Think about the last time you acted out of envy or scarcity. The last time you withheld praise because you thought giving it would somehow take something from you. Too often in our careers, we deprive others of well-deserved recognition because we believe it will detract from our value. I've been guilty of doing it too.

A few years back, I read an excerpt from *A New Earth: Awakening to Your Life's Purpose* by author Eckhart Tolle, and the truth landed like a bucket of cold water. It was a spiritual interruption I didn't know I needed, and it changed my attitude forever:

> *People unknowingly sabotage their own work when they withhold help or information from others or try to undermine them lest they become more successful or get more credit than "me." The ego doesn't know that the more you include others, the more smoothly things flow and the more easily things come to you. When you give little or no help to others or put obstacles in their path, the universe—in the form of people and circumstances—gives little or no help to you because you have cut yourself off from the whole. . . . You cannot receive what you don't give. Outflow determines Inflow. Whatever you think the world is withholding from you, you already have, but unless you allow it to flow out, you won't know that you have it. This is the source of Abundance.*[2]

So, give the praise. Open the door and pass the ladder down. Choose abundance every time, because what you give will flow back. But only if you let it out first.

Faith Echoes

#1: Being a good Christian doesn't mean keeping the peace no matter the cost.

I used to think that being a "good Christian" in the workplace meant staying quiet, keeping the peace, turning the other cheek, and never complaining when the slap left a bruise. I chose peace over punishment and silence over disruption. But that isn't forgiveness; that's the silent degradation of your self-worth.

Forgiveness begins when there is the intention to repair. But allowing someone to repeatedly inflict harm through bullying, exclusion, or passive aggression and calling it grace? That's not faith. That's spiritual bypassing. Because toxicity isn't only a personal wound; it's a workplace infection. And when it's left to fester, it corrodes both the victim and the culture.

God never asked us to be gullible. He said:

Matthew 10:16: *"Be wise as serpents, and innocent as doves" (ESV).*

Wisdom and forgiveness are not the same thing. Yes, offer the other cheek. But when harm becomes a pattern—deliberate, repeated, destructive—letting go without boundaries is not holiness; it's self-erasure. God does not call us to that. Learn the difference. Stand up for yourself in courage, confidence, and grace.

#2: One of the best feelings for a believer is "Retrospective Gratitude."

When I think about my rejections, I realize that if they hadn't happened, I wouldn't have been led here. I often contemplate one of the most sacred feelings as a believer, which I call "retrospective gratitude." It doesn't arrive in the moment when everything is breaking, when life at work or home is tough, not when your prayers feel like they're hitting brick ceilings, and certainly not when you're clutching your dreams in one hand and watching them crumble through the other. It takes days, months, and sometimes years, but one morning or midnight hour, you will look back and whisper, "*Thank You, God, for not giving me what I asked fo*r."

I used to stand in prayer, sometimes performatively, begging God: *Let Your will be done.* But buried beneath that prayer, stitched deep into my pleading, was this quiet translation: *If You really love me like You say, then please let it go my way.* I'm now unspeakably grateful those prayers went unanswered. Because if they had gone my way, I don't think I would have gone on this wild, uncharted pursuit of purpose. I wouldn't have knocked on unconventional doors or built new ones from splintered hope after the familiar ones slammed shut in my face.

I had to learn (and relearn) that trusting God is easy when the metrics say you're winning. When the manager is pleased, the patients are grateful, the projects are gaining traction, and your career graph is on an upward trajectory. But what about when everything halts?

What happens when all the doors close? When the vision unravels faster than you can patch it? When the calling feels heavier than you can carry, lonelier than you imagined, and completely unrewarded? When your life or your career looks nothing like the success story you rehearsed in your head? That's when trust becomes more than a word. It becomes oxygen, a lifeline for your unraveling soul.

Jeremiah 29:11: *"For I know the plans I have for you," declares the* LORD. *"Plans to prosper you and not to harm you, plans to give you hope and a future."*

There were seasons when I clung to that verse because it was the only thing I had left to hold on to. Everything else felt unstable, uncertain, and unfair. But His plan is always intact, even when mine falls to pieces. And somehow, clinging to that verse made room for grace.

You may be reading this in the midst of your own unraveling. Maybe your job is gone, your title feels hollow, or the version of life you built is crumbling. But please hear this: The end of your plan does not mean the end of His plan.

You are not forgotten. And those unanswered prayers are not rejections. They are redirections wrapped in mercy. Hold on, even if the path ahead is overgrown, the silence feels unbearable, and your voice shakes every time you say, "I still trust You." Because when the dust settles and the new story emerges, trust me, you will be grateful. Not instantly, but in holy, retrospective clarity. The kind that only the believer understands.

Unscript Yourself Toolkit

Permission to Shine Your Brilliance

Come as you are. No productivity guilt; this is calibration.
One true line per prompt is better than ten perfect ones.

What bullying warning signs have you brushed aside in a workplace out of fear, uncertainty, or pressure to keep the peace?

____

____

____

Have you ever dimmed your excellence to make others more comfortable? What did it cost you?

____

____

____

Can you recall a moment when your vigilance changed the course of a patient's care? How did that moment impact you?

____

____

____

Unscripted Permission Slips

- You have permission to be excellent and stop dimming your brilliance to keep fragile egos comfortable. Your light is meant to illuminate, not shrink to protect someone else's comfort.
- You have permission to name bullying for what it is, even when everyone else minimizes it. Silence is not loyalty; it is self-erasure.
- You have permission to trust your vigilance, your instinct, your "something feels off" intuition. That nudge is your clinical wisdom speaking.

Unscripted Affirmation

My excellence is not arrogance,
and my vigilance is not rebellion;
they are my obedience to my Call to More,
and I will not shrink from them.

PART IV

The Awakening

"You didn't plan on each day looking the same, did you? In a job that might be smothering your soul. Dealing with stressful worries and endless responsibilities that stifle your originality and steal your energy."

—ROBIN SHARMA, THE 5 AM CLUB

CHAPTER 8

You Have What It Takes

Deep down, you know what you want and have what it takes.

—Maxime Legace

It was another solo Saturday shift, the kind that demanded head-down automation that didn't bend under the load. I remember looking up from the dispensary; the script queue stretched like a never-ending scroll, and thinking, *God, these solo shifts have shaped me enough. I can't keep working like a pressure cooker.*

It wasn't just the workload. It was the feeling that I was a threat to someone else that gave me extreme discomfort. He'd said it out loud once, and I'd seen how quickly things could spiral when egos were bruised in the pharmacy world. How revenge could masquerade as policy, and how feedback could be twisted into insubordination. I wanted out before things got ugly—again!

But here's the thing: I also felt guilty for wanting more. Deeply, irrationally guilty. People around me (friends, colleagues, family) reminded me how lucky I was to have a job at all. They'd say things like, "Be grateful you have a job that pays the bills. It's secure."

Never mind that it paid those bills with forty-hour workweeks, no weekends, and missed milestones in my kids' lives. Or that I went home every night hollow-eyed and spiritually starved. I often wondered if maybe they were right. Maybe I should silence the voice inside, the one whispering, *This isn't it,* and learn to be content.

But that voice wouldn't go quiet. It wasn't an entitled voice. It felt honest. It wasn't asking for escape but alignment. Still, I said nothing because the guilt of wanting more was so internalized that I didn't realize I was holding myself hostage to it.

The guilt of wanting more was so internalized that I didn't realize I was holding myself hostage to it.

I've always been someone who sees things first in pictures—a mental blueprinting I've leaned on again and again throughout my career when I encounter problems and want to create solutions. So, I began the quiet but determined hunt for a workplace that might finally recognize, or at least not suppress, the potential I knew I carried. I wasn't just looking for a different job; I was searching for a place that would allow me to expand, to step beyond the counter's constraints and practice pharmacy as I had always imagined: a hub of clinical services rooted in relationship and purpose, where value-based care wasn't an afterthought but the foundation.

As if the vision I was holding had rippled beyond my mind, life threw me a curious thread. My husband and I were building a house in a new suburb when, on a weekend drive past the dusty plot that would someday become our home, I noticed something: a new complex rising from the earth, sitting oddly in the middle of an otherwise uninhabited stretch of land.

I remember saying it out loud, more as a wish than a statement, "I wonder what's going on in there. Imagine if it were a medical center with a pharmacy."

A couple of weeks later, I saw a job listing. A position opened at a pharmacy, and the owner was a pharmacist from my peer group—someone who knew my work ethic. I reached out to her, and after a series of long conversations, she offered me a better position than the one listed. She invited me to join her new pharmacy. This wasn't just any pharmacy; it was one at that same site I'd driven past, the one I'd half-prayed into possibility without realizing it.

After all the years of pushing to bloom in spaces that offered no sunlight, this felt like a divine yes—an opportunity almost too generous to believe. For the first time in my career, I truly felt acknowledged. My vision didn't have to be explained, diluted, or justified—it was welcomed. The owner believed in what I saw and encouraged it. This was the clean slate I'd prayed for, a chance to take everything I'd imagined in the quiet moments, every unconventional idea, every clinical dream deferred, and build something real.

A few months passed in that dreamy limbo of possibility before the pharmacy officially opened and the first shift began. I stepped into the role of pharmacy manager, tasked with overseeing a brand-new space, collaborating with doctors and allied health professionals, and helping shape the clinical culture from day one.

Little did I know that new businesses are slow to find their rhythm, and for the first few months, the patient database barely trickled in. The pressure to keep things running fell squarely on me. Eventually, patients started flowing in, prescriptions began piling up, and the pharmacy was beginning to "succeed" by every external metric. But instead of relief, I felt a familiar suffocation creeping back in. Working solo while the prescription volume was growing, I found myself another cog in the wheel, spinning endlessly with no time to pause, no chance to talk with patients, and no space for offering the care I'd once imagined this role would allow.

Once again, *This isn't what I signed up for.* I remember thinking one afternoon as I stood behind the counter, back aching, brain fogged, eyes scanning yet another stack of repeats. What I love about being a pharmacist is the meaningful interactions that impact patients. I could do with less time pumping out four hundred-plus prescriptions a day solo, feeling like a dementor is sucking the living hell out of me. (I also wish someone had warned me that getting to the toilet would become an eight-hour mission.)

The resentment rose not toward others, but toward myself. I was ashamed of daring to believe this system would ever make room for my vision. I grew frustrated that I'd let myself get hopeful, that I'd once again convinced myself it would be different this time. Maybe I had unrealistic expectations. And, as one does, I entered an endless cycle of gaslighting myself.

Eventually, I did what I always do when the hope frays: I tried to fix it. I shared my struggle with the owner. I was burned out from working alone. I explained how my clinical ideas were collecting dust, how the day-to-day grind was eroding the purpose I'd come here to pursue. But her answer was the one I'd heard before, only wrapped in a more compassionate tone: "We can't sustain hiring another pharmacist."

And that was the moment the truth settled in heavier than any script load. After a decade in this field—job after job, vision after vision—I finally understood my reality: *This is it.* This is what pharmacy has become: a model dictated by funding, not by patients, and certainly not by pharmacists. The creative vision I had brought to the table—the clinical services, the innovative workflows, the reimagining of what pharmacy could look like—was crushed under the relentless pressure of dispensing. I was stuck, again! Only this time, I had exhausted every opportunity I knew how to chase.

Naturally, disappointment hovered, but I knew I couldn't afford to spiral. So instead of giving in to it, I redirected my energy and poured what little I had into the one thing that still gave me meaning: connecting with my patients.

In the rare moments when it wasn't too busy, I focused on building strong patient relationships and offering care that felt human, generous, and personal. I made follow-up calls. I took the time, when it was available, to establish connections. Slowly, word-of-mouth referrals started coming in. Ironically, it was this forced pivot that became the pinnacle of everything I'd later build. That chapter taught me more about business building, customer experience, stock management, and interprofessional collaboration than any MBA ever could.

As if the universe knew I was running on fumes, the jolt of motivation I'd been gasping for arrived right on cue. The Pharmaceutical Society of New Zealand (PSNZ) announced an opportunity for early-career pharmacists (ECPs) to apply for sponsorship to attend the Pharmaceutical Society of Australia's conference in Sydney in 2018. I've never shied away from opportunity, and if I could shout from every dispensary rooftop, "Fortune favors the bold!" I would. Embracing the Unscripted journey means having the courage to lean into opportunity. If you don't show up for enough noes, you'll never get the yes that rearranges your entire trajectory. And though I had my fair share of rejections, when it came to opportunities that mattered, God knew I was unrelenting and mercifully aligned things in my favor.

► PRO-TIP

Don't just attend conferences that top up your clinical knowledge. Seek out events with varied, future-focused themes: innovation, systems-thinking, mindset, and cross-sector collaboration. These are the conferences that set you apart in your career.

Alongside a few other ECPs, we headed off to Sydney, and that experience was nothing short of enlightening. I needed the connection with colleagues after months of working in isolation. It was healing. What I absorbed in those conference rooms wasn't just CPD; it was the networking, the exposure, the speakers, and the shared energy of ambitious pharmacists from every corner of the globe. It was empowering. The right conference feeds not only your mind; it expands your thinking, shifts your posture, teaches you to innovate, and makes you bolder in how you show up in the workplace.

Upon my return from the conference, our small cohort of ECPs felt something stir. We had seen firsthand the advocacy work being done by our Australian counterparts, and the contrast was impossible to ignore. There was a noticeable gap in how ECPs were supported, particularly in working conditions, leadership development, and access to real career-building opportunities.

A few of us who attended the conference were appointed to the Early-Career Pharmacist Steering Group, where we led the development of the PSNZ Early-Career Pharmacist Building Blocks Report, a landmark document outlining ten recommendations for action to better support ECPs across New Zealand. It was the first time I saw what advocacy could do—not in theory or policy, but in real time. I tucked the experience under my belt, unaware it was laying track for the next step.

That experience, combined with my appointment to the Pharmacy

Council Professional Conduct Committee a few years earlier, formed a sturdy enough foundation—one that would eventually lead to something I never saw coming: my appointment to the Board of the Pharmacy Council of New Zealand (PCNZ). And it all began, as many defining moments do, in the most unremarkable way.

A few months after our ECP Building Blocks Report was published, I was casually flipping through a *Pharmacy Today* magazine when I came across a call for expressions of interest in joining the PCNZ board. The application deadline was five p.m. that same day. I glanced at the clock: four p.m. And in what can only be described as a moment of panic and boldness, I threw together a half-baked application and hit send without ceremony. No vision board. No expectation of hearing back. Of course, I included everything and anything that might signal leadership, advocacy, or a heartbeat for the profession. I stretched my CV like a rubber band, hoping it wouldn't snap. I thought, *Well, if I get declined, at least I gave it a go.* I forgot about it for eight months.

It was August 2019, eight months after my last-minute application, when the unexpected call came on a stressful workday. I picked up the phone to a lady saying, "Hi, it's X from the Ministry of Health. Is Katrina there?" Then there was silence. My brain froze. I was freaking out. Every neuron in my brain screamed: *Oh no! What have I done?* What felt like a pause of about five seconds was a lifetime when the lady finally interrupted, saying, "Hello, are you there?" I responded with no greeting, just a blunt, fearful, "Yes, what have I done?" "You have done nothing. I am calling to inform you that the Minister of Health has appointed you to the Pharmacy Council of New Zealand board," she responded.

That's when I broke down hysterically into tears of relief more than joy. It was the relief to find out I wasn't being held accountable for any wrongdoing. The relief that I wasn't in trouble. That this wasn't another accusation, another inquiry, or another moment of professional vulnerability; it was sad that my brain didn't register

► **PRO-TIP**

When applying for jobs, never underestimate the value of the things you've done quietly, locally, or from the heart. That community event you helped run, the grassroots advocacy group you showed up for, leading that Sunday school class at church. They're not footnotes. They are proof of your humanity. Decision-makers are looking for humans, not robots.

celebration in that moment. It only registered danger.

► **PRO-TIP**

Don't wait until you feel ready. Just put forward the hidden work you've already done, even if it feels small and imperfect. Trust that consistency builds credibility over time.

Yet somehow, I had been appointed. I would be the youngest member at the board table. People often say, "You got lucky." But I don't believe in luck. I believe in being prepared when the door opens. In doing the hidden work that nobody sees. In putting yourself out there, even when it feels clumsy or premature. And in seeking the truest, most aligned expression of yourself in everything you do. If anything made that moment possible, it was rejection familiarity: years of unanswered emails and ghosted applications, with some quiet noes and some brutal ones. I became immune to rejection, and that immunity became my superpower. It can be yours, too, if you let it, because no application is ever wasted; it's all resistance training.

Too many pharmacists early in their careers let fear become a full stop. They hesitate, overthink, delay, and quietly disqualify themselves long before anyone else has the chance to recognize their potential. But fear is standing between you and your potential, and the only way through is to leap anyway.

This chapter in my career is a badge of honor I hold with deep gratitude because it changed me. Serving on the Pharmacy Council board has been one the most humbling learning curves I've encountered. Most pharmacists have no idea how challenging this role can be, and I don't blame you; I didn't either. Like you, I once believed the work was primarily symbolic, strategic, and bureaucratic. But regulation, I've come to learn, is layered and often misunderstood. I don't think I truly grasped its complexity until a year or more into the role. At first, I assumed I was stepping into a position of advocacy, serving as a voice for the profession. But deep mentorship and hard-won insight taught me that regulation ensures competence, upholds professional standards, and ensures patient safety.

Pharmacy is a demanding profession, and I see it reflected in the complaints we review around the Council table. I see young pharmacists, many starting their careers, making poor decisions that lead to irreversible consequences. Sometimes it's burnout or pressure, and sometimes it's isolation and fear. This is the part of the board role I struggle with most. By the time the complaints arrive, it's already too late. By the time a pharmacist is sitting in front of the Health and Disability Commissioner, their world has often already crumbled. And all I can think is: *I wish I could have reached them sooner. I wish someone had told them the truth before they made that mistake or poor decision. I wish I could have been the voice in the dark saying,* "You're not alone. Don't let the system break you before you ask for help."

That's why I'm sharing this now, openly and honestly, without polish or pretense. If one person reading this seeks support instead of suffering in silence, if one person asks for help instead of making that costly, career-altering decision, this chapter was worth writing.

Unscript Yourself Echoes

#1: Gratitude isn't a gag order.

Society confuses ambition with ingratitude. And the cost? We murder potential. We slaughter talent. We crucify creativity.

Let me clarify the distinction: ingratitude is a chronic state of complaining. It's the mindset that refuses to see good anywhere—in work and in everyday life. It is the "glass is always half-empty" instead of "half-full" attitude. But wanting more from your career? Wanting to grow, to contribute more, to offer more, to make an impact? That isn't ingratitude; that is ambition.

We rarely talk about it, but many pharmacists carry this quiet ache. It's the belief that dissatisfaction makes us unworthy. If the job pays well, then we should be silent. If we have some stability, then we have no right to dream.

The problem is that we live in a world that punishes audacity and suppresses talent and creativity. Even though we have come a long way in the last decade, the guilt of wanting more lingers and is often so internalized that we cannot overcome it. But here is what I understand: *Gratitude and growth are not enemies.* You can honor the season that sustained you *and* outgrow it. You can bless the job that fed your family *and* say, "This no longer fits." You can give thanks for the opportunity *and still* walk away when your soul shrinks.

The truth is, your vision is not ungrateful. It is evidence that your spirit is still alive.

#2: Dial out of disappointment.

Disappointment is an ugly beast when it rears its head. It is bad enough when you are disappointed in others, but when you are disappointed in yourself, it is agonizing. You cannot change others, so you eventually let go, but when it comes to yourself, the voice of beratement is unrelenting. There are many times when the vision you are striving for does not come to life the way you imagined.

Disappointment hits hard when expectations do not meet reality. Work-related disappointment is one of the worst; after all, that is where you spend most of your day. You walk into that new job with fire in your bones, ready to build, change things, and finally feel useful. After a while, you find yourself stuck again, pouring metrics instead of purpose. And when that happens, you have two choices: you can either spiral into bitterness or shift your focus to what you *can* control—not in a toxic positivity way, but in a grounded, clarity-seeking way.

So, you redirect your energy. You find the micro-moments where you *can* make an impact. You choose excellence, even in unseen places, and you offer presence and build trust in the quiet corners of a noisy system. Eventually, the practice of integrity—not perfection or productivity—becomes your anchor. You may not change the system today, but you *can* change how you show up in it, and sometimes that's where the real shift begins.

#3: Stop chasing credentials and start believing in your worth.

The people who change systems aren't always the most qualified, but they're often the most willing. They're the ones who say, "I've seen the gap, and I can't unsee it." They're the ones who don't wait for someone else to take initiative. They may not get recognized for it at first, but eventually, they will. Choose to be the one to lead with initiative. You don't need a title to lead. You need lived experience, a little audacity, and a refusal to wait for permission because the reality is you will never be given it.

Your next level isn't found in the script you've been handed. It is hiding behind an application sent in fear of rejection. You often wait for signs, for qualifications, and for confidence, but what you truly need is to believe in your worth. It isn't about how polished you feel; it's about the willingness to leap before you're ready because you will never be ready enough.

I was never qualified "enough" for almost every position I applied for, but I applied anyway. If I had known what boxes I was supposed to tick, I probably would have ticked them all and still felt unworthy. Though you may not tick all the boxes, your courage to change the narrative, if true, will draw the right outcome to you. Some people call this type of attitude passion; I call it chasing purpose, impact, and legacy.

Faith Echoes

#1: When the doors close, you must trust God, do what's right, and choose optimism.

This is one of the hardest things to live out, and I say that not as someone who mastered it early, but as someone who had to learn it the long, painful way. When the doors close, especially at work, where so much of your time, energy, and identity can feel entangled, it's tempting to let cynicism take the wheel.

To say, "Forget it. I'm done." To walk away in bitterness, to shrink back, to settle for half-hearted effort because the system doesn't deserve your excellence. But here's what I've learned to do instead:

1. **Trust God.**
   Even when it doesn't make sense. Even when your prayers feel unheard. Even when you're angry, heart-weary, and secretly wondering if you misread the whole calling in the first place. Trust God. Trust doesn't always look like bold declarations. Sometimes it's about quiet obedience and staying the course one more day.

2. **Do what's right.**
   Don't do what's easiest. Don't react. Don't give in to what your emotions scream for. Continue to show up with integrity, to speak truth with grace, and to work as if your labor is seen, even if no one applauds. Every unseen act of faithfulness is recorded in heaven's ledgers—not on social media and certainly not by your boss. I say this because I've lived it. We often do the right thing, hoping quietly that someone, especially the boss, will notice; that they will reward our efforts and see how valuable we are behind our silence. But when that recognition doesn't come, it can wound you more than the original disappointment ever did. And that's when trust becomes sacred. That's when faith becomes the only fuel left in the tank.
3. **Choose optimism over pessimism.**
   Choosing optimism does not mean projecting toxic positivity or delusion, but hope grounded in Christ. The spirit-fed hope that whispers, *God is in control.* Choosing optimism is not about ignoring reality but anchoring your heart in a deeper one. It's saying, "This is hard, but it won't always be this hard. And God is still good even here."

   It's difficult to do this. I've had many moments when I wanted to burn it all down—quit, escape, numb out, start over. But in hindsight, I've learned that a positive attitude, consistent integrity, and an unwavering trust in God have always attracted the right opportunities back to me. Not immediately, and certainly not on my timeline, but eventually, they always did!

Galatians 6:9: *"Let us not become weary in doing good, for at the proper time we will reap a harvest if we do not give up."*

#2: God doesn't call the qualified. He qualifies the called.

If I've learned anything in my career journey, it's that God doesn't call the qualified; He qualifies the called. He chooses the people with messy résumés, shattered confidence, and unfiltered prayers. He chooses the unlikely, the overlooked, the "not quite ready." And when He calls for you, you will often feel the most underprepared you've ever felt. But that's the point, because then you have no choice but to rely on Him. You will walk with reverence, not ego, and make room for miracles.

Every time I stepped into something that felt bigger than me—some boardroom, stage, "writing a book," or responsibility I didn't feel qualified for—I saw His hand carry what my credentials could not. The favor didn't follow the degree; it followed my obedience, my faith, and my belief that I was stepping into the dream He had for me when He created me. I stepped into His purpose for my life.

So, if you're standing at the threshold, convinced you're not enough, remember: God doesn't ask for your perfection. He asks for your trust in Him to step into His purpose for you. He asks you to step into His grace.

2 Corinthians 12:9: *"But he said to me, 'My grace is sufficient for you, for my power is made perfect in weakness.' Therefore, I will boast all the more gladly about my weaknesses, so that Christ's power may rest on me."*

Unscript Yourself Toolkit

Permission to Believe You're Already Qualified

Show up human, not heroic. One honest scrawl is worth more than ten overworked answers.

Can you recall a time you felt guilty for wanting more, when that guilt was so internalized that you began to gaslight yourself? If it happened again today, how might you handle it differently?

____

____

____

What opportunity or application are you talking yourself out of because you don't feel ready? What would pressing send look like this week?

____

____

____

Think of one career disappointment you've faced. How could you reframe it as training instead of failure?

____

____

____

Unscripted Permission Slips

- You have permission to want more without calling it ingratitude.
- You have permission to honor the job that sustained you and still outgrow it.
- You have permission to believe you already carry what it takes for the next step.

Unscripted Affirmation

I am allowed to want more; every "no" has trained me for the "yes" that will shift my story, and I already have what it takes.

CHAPTER 9

You Are Not Broken: You Are a Human and a Healer

Nothing in healthcare is so healing as the human touch. That's what patients need most.

—Katrina Azer

Our accessibility is our greatest strength, but on some days, it can also be our greatest weakness. No one understands the toll all the demands take on your mental health as a community pharmacist until you've faced a harrowing situation.

It happened on another busy weekday—chaotic and fast-paced. But the events of that day did more than hurt my feelings; they broke me. It was the day a patient physically assaulted me.

He was one of my regulars, the kind you know by name, who often tests your patience. He was a lovely man but had a touch of volatility. One day, he stormed into the dispensary mid-mayhem, slammed his hands on the counter, and barked, "Where is my insulin?"

I paused, taken aback. I couldn't recall dispensing anything for him recently. I searched his record. Nothing. "I'm sorry, Mr. X," I said gently. "I can't see anything from the doctor yet."

"All right," he growled, pacing. "I'll call them and come back in an hour." He then stormed out.

An hour later, he returned, acting even more agitated and unpredictable. It was a Friday afternoon, and you know what that means. It's like you are in a war zone rather than a pharmacy.

Uh-oh, he looks angrier than before, I thought. I took a few steps toward him, trying to preempt another eruption. "I'm really sorry, Mr. X," I said. "We still haven't received anything from the doctor."

In that moment, all hell broke loose. The next thing I knew, he grabbed my arm (suddenly, tightly, violently), and before I could process it, he flung me into the consultation room and slammed the door shut behind us. Then he went ballistic. I don't remember what he said—something about how it was my fault his script wasn't ready and how I had wasted his day. The pain in my arm was burning through my sleeve. My mind had shifted from professional to primal as I fought the rising panic. I wasn't listening to him, which only made the situation worse. Had I been listening and responding, perhaps he would've calmed down. Instead, I was strategizing how to get out of the darn room safely. Scared of what he might do next, I prayed a prayer that someone about to die might've prayed. Thankfully, other waiting patients had been watching this madness unfold, and one of them opened the door within seconds, but those seconds felt like hours. She pointed her finger at him, admonished him for treating a staff member as such, and told him to let me go immediately.

I headed back to the dispensary with my face down, trying my best to hold it together. But I couldn't, and I eventually broke down quietly while still dispensing the last few prescriptions of the day, hanging on until six p.m. And by "last few," I mean about eighty more. Because that's how pharmacy works: you're allowed to shatter, but only once the queue is cleared!

I kept smiling back at patients with tearful, crooked smiles while ducking behind the dispensary pillar so patients wouldn't see the full force of the breakdown forming behind my eyes. My retail team member tried to console me, whispering gentle words while I robotically scanned barcodes, labeled boxes, answered the phone, and handed out meds. Some patients who witnessed the incident stared at me from behind the counter, wondering how I was still functioning.

One of them said I should've called the police. In that moment, the healer in me couldn't bear to turn a human crisis into a criminal scene. I wanted de-escalation, not punishment. But experience has since taught me not to confuse compassion with the absence of boundaries or mercy with the suspension of safety. Calling for help is how we protect every life in the room, including our own. I've since learned that calling for help is neither a betrayal of my calling nor an act of betrayal toward a patient. Calling for help and holding those who act violently accountable are required to uphold the profession's fidelity.

I made it to the last prescription, and the grill doors finally came down. Then I sat on the floor and sobbed my fear and hurt out. The shock had been contained for the last hour, but now it leaked out in uncontrollable tears. I wasn't experiencing frustration or anger, but fear—and immense disappointment in the system that allowed this to happen. If the doctor had understood that the diabetic patient needed his meds so urgently, it would not have culminated in my abuse.

I called the pharmacy owner and told her what happened. We agreed to issue a trespass notice—meaning he was formally banned from entering the pharmacy again—not out of revenge or retribution, but because I was genuinely afraid of what might happen if he came back. The thought of seeing that patient again sent chills down my spine.

That Friday evening sob, those quiet tears behind the counter, became the moment that made me let go. I felt so unsafe at my job that I started building the quiet momentum to leave. Something had changed. Forever this time.

And yet, it wasn't all devastation. I still love community pharmacy. Because for every soul-crushing moment you encounter, there are sacred ones too. Moments that remind you why you show up in the first place. We give people space, time, and, most of all, our presence. Even when we're pressed against the wall with scripts, shortages, and phone calls, we still try to pause long enough to listen, and that listening creates a bond that's deeper than many other encounters in healthcare.

One of the understated beauties of working in a small, tight-knit community is how intimately you come to know your patients—their children, their stories, and, sadly, the ones we become so well acquainted with that when a tragic diagnosis arrives and their health spirals, the watching becomes its own agony.

I won't pretend that I always held the line. There were a few times my empathy broke open into full-blown grief. I've cried with patients' families at the counter, especially in those sacred, painful moments when they walk in holding the bag of leftover morphine ampoules—bags we know too well—because we've followed their loved one's journey for months, knowing that final day would soon come. The day they bring the bag of unwanted meds—*the bag that signals the end.*

And there you'd be, standing at the counter, the eyes of the caregiver (be it a husband, wife, son, or daughter) piercing through you, silently begging for someone who could meet their grief with more than polite condolences. Someone who knew. Who had witnessed the decline. Who had spoken softly through the pain, who remembered.

I'm crying as I write this because I can still see one of those patients in my mind—one of the loveliest patients I've ever met. So gentle and gracious. Even after he received his terminal diagnosis, he still smiled and checked in on each team member. Over the course of six months, I watched that smile fade. First, he stopped coming in; then his wife began collecting the meds. Until one day, she came in with the bag. The bag of palliative care meds that every time I dispose of, I'm reminded of how short life is. She fell into my arms and sobbed hysterically. I couldn't find any words, so I cried with her.

They taught us at pharmacy school to maintain boundaries: to empathize but not sympathize. But the human in me couldn't do that. I cried because I, too, felt the weight of the loss of a patient I had seen almost every other day. Of someone who showed me care, even as his own life was slipping away. Of someone whose final months were managed by the medication I dispensed, the smile I offered, the questions I bothered to ask in a system that so often rushed them out the door.

And then there were the elderly patients and the war veterans who treated the pharmacy like their daily outing. They dressed up, came to the pharmacy, and waited patiently just to be seen and interact with a familiar face.

Mr. Smith (pseudonym) was one of those people. He used to come in and tell me about his wife, who had Alzheimer's and had forgotten who he was. He had cared for her faithfully for over thirty years, yet she didn't know him anymore. He told me all that with tears quietly swelling in his eyes. One day, I asked him gently, "You live so far away. Why do you come all the way here?" He looked at me and said, with a trembling, tearful whisper, "Because you're a familiar face who cares. My wife doesn't know who I am. My kids haven't checked on me in years, but you do. You make sure I've got the right meds, that nothing is missing from my script. You check to see how I'm coping. No one else does that. Not even my doctor. That's why I come here. Because you care." His words were so impactful that they made me tear up. And that, my friends, is the meaning of community pharmacy.

And let's not forget about all the meaningful interventions we never talk about because we're too damn tired, or should I say we're too used to fixing the system's near-fatal mistakes. Interventions like the methotrexate 20 mg daily prescription.

It was on one of those pre–long weekend shifts, and amid the chaos, I received a script for methotrexate 20 mg daily. My fried brain entered the data through the system, clicking through alert after alert. (You know those days when you keep hitting "OK" without reading a single thing? Yeah, that was me.) I got to the dispensing bench, slapped the label on, and paused.

Wait, what? Daily? Why is that daily?

If you've ever stared at a dose that made your stomach sink and still hesitated to pick up the phone to double-check it with the doctor, you're not incompetent; you're human in a hierarchy, which can be intimidating.

I called the doctor's receptionist, who passed me to the nurse, who was no help and promised the doctor would call me back. The patient was anxious to head away for the weekend. Two hours went by, but still no call. I called the doctor myself to explain what was happening, and he cut me off with, "Yes, I saw it. That's the correct dose." *Click.*

No space for discussion. No pause. Just a prescription that, as far as I knew, was sending an urgent request to the angels to pick up the patient's soul.

So I did what any stubborn, fed-up pharmacist would do: I walked across to the medical center. My emotions hissed, *Are you sure you want to push his buttons?* But my logic was louder: *You have an ethical duty to prevent harm.* His door was open (a small mercy).

"Dr. X, are you really sure—"

"Yes, I said it was correct," he interrupted.

Without letting him finish, I raised my tone—sharp, loud, deliberate. "You prescribed twenty milligrams—as in two-zero—daily. Is that your intention?"

He paused for a moment before answering. "What? Not daily."

"Well, that's what you've got here."

"I didn't mean that. It's weekly."

"Well, that's what I've been trying to establish for the last six hours, and the patient is getting increasingly frustrated with me."

"Oh, no! I'm sorry. That isn't what I meant. I'll reprint the script with the correct dose."

Thank God for pharmacists!

Then there are the prescriptions so dubious you hold the label in one hand and your license in the other, questioning the prescriber's judgment while your courage hides behind your teeth. You don't dare to call because power dynamics are real. I've been there.

I recall two patients, a woman and her partner, who would each come in every Friday with a prescription for Ritalin 20 mg SR, three tablets, *three times a day.* I dispensed them every week, and each time I felt a dull ache screaming inside me. It didn't look right. It didn't feel right. But it came from a specialist, so surely he knew what he was doing, right?

I called to confirm the dose when I filled them for the first time. I couldn't find any clinical references to justify the dose. Still, the doctor approved it. One Friday, the woman came alone to get both scripts filled. I decided that time that I'd had enough of dispensing these prescriptions when every instinct I had was not to, so I told her we were busy and that the prescriptions would be ready in forty-five minutes (call it a white lie in the interest of public safety).

In that pause, I turned over every stone. I called another psychiatrist. I phoned our pharmacy association's practice support team. I reached out to doctor friends. I asked other pharmacists. No one thought that dose was clinically appropriate. I rang the Medical Council. They agreed I should file a report. My moral and ethical duty was wrestling with fear, throwing up reservations—*He's a psychiatrist. Who are you to challenge this?*—while another voice rose to meet it: *Your signature is going on this. Your scope includes exercising clinical judgment, and you can't un-know what you know now.*

I wrote a note on the prescription: "Not dispensed because of concerns with clinical appropriateness."

When she came back to collect them, I calmly explained I wouldn't be dispensing the medication. The woman snatched the prescriptions and bolted out the door. A few months later, I found out that the psychiatrist's registration had been revoked.

These are our untold stories, and no doubt you have many. The stories you carry silently about impact, safety, and connection that you never share. The stories that get buried under society's expectations and by systems that no longer focus on connection and prevention, but on transaction, volume, and compliance checklists that reduce your care to metrics on a dashboard. And so the moments that matter—the counseling that calmed a patient's fear, the intervention that averted harm, the quiet presence that reminded a patient they were seen—fade into the background, unrecorded, unnamed, and uncelebrated. Yet these are the very stories that prove you are more than the script and more than the silence that tries to swallow you whole.

This is what community pharmacists do every day and never get credit for. We prevent harm in our communities, and we seldom get thanked for it. You are not just a medication dispenser or counseling point; you are a healer in your community. That's why I chose to be the catalyst to build recognition for our role, to put system boundaries that protect pharmacists, and to empower pharmacists to own their future and tap into the Call to More.

You are not just a medication dispenser or counseling point; you are a healer in your community.

Unscript Yourself Echoes

The quiet power of the Pharmacist.

I wonder how many pharmacists reading this can relate to some form of patient aggression. Maybe not physical, but a sharp tongue, a pointed accusation, an angry outburst hurled your way on a day when you were already stretched thin.

Early in my career, I used to take it personally. Their frustration would pierce straight through me, and I'd wear it like a badge of failure. But over time, I came to understand something deeper about healthcare and its tangled systems. Patients don't mean to aim their arrows at us; it's because we are often the last in the chain—the only accessible human in a system that has failed them over and over again.

What they often need isn't a perfect solution but someone to listen with an engaged presence. Not the cold, clinical "uh-huh" while typing, but the kind of listening that makes them feel seen. A listening that says, *I know you're hurting. I'm not the one who caused it, but I won't disappear.*

Unfortunately, it's when you get the rare chaotic ones that throw you off, and you're expected to carry on afterward as if nothing happened, even if the wound wasn't physical, when it was just words flung in a moment of rage. But words hurt. They humiliate you, destabilize your focus, and dissolve your sense of safety. Even so, you're expected to return to the counter, to keep going like you didn't just get emotionally battered. But you weren't made to endure the unendurable because you're a "health professional."

These are the moments when the healers need healing. And the cruelest part? The support channels are so scarce, so tangled in bureaucracy that sometimes there's no one to turn to. No one to say, "Are you okay?"

No space to admit that your concentration has been hijacked, your nervous system shaken, and your sense of self temporarily shattered. I know there are practitioner support programs, and I encourage you to explore them if you can, but asking for help in extreme moments isn't easy. It never felt easy for me. I was too ashamed to admit the hurt. But if you've been there—or if you're there now—I see you. I feel it with you. And I want you to hear this loud and clear: You are not broken. The system you work in is. You are, and will always be, the respected healthcare professional your community needs. Don't let one (or more) acts of violence, cruelty, or misdirected rage dictate your worth, your calling, or your future.

There's a difference between being "just the dispenser" and being the reason someone stays alive. Sometimes we forget what it means to be a pharmacist. Pharmacists catch fatal errors every day—often alone, often unseen, often without the support or acknowledgment they deserve.

We're trained to follow protocols, obey authority, and assume that if a doctor signs it, then it must be right. But we're not just the middle people; we're the last line of defense in a system that still treats us like glorified vending machines.

We double-check. We take the fall for the errors we didn't make. We're the ones who catch the dose that could kill. The ones who say, "Wait, this doesn't feel right," and actually act on it. We don't just hand out meds; we interrogate them. We don't just trust systems; we challenge them. And in doing so, we save lives that may never thank us, and we prevent harm that no one else saw coming.

This is advocacy in action. It's more than professionalism. It's purpose. That's what makes a pharmacist more than a title. It's what makes us indispensable, even if the system forgets our true value. That is the quiet power of the pharmacist.

Faith Echoes

God wants your fearful whispers and trembling heart.

Amidst fear, remembering to turn to God for help is often the last thing we do. When the amygdala takes over, our breath shortens, our bodies tense, and our emotions scream, while faith becomes almost nonexistent. Ironically, it is in those moments when the mind goes to war with itself that we need God the most.

In that consultation room, I didn't remember to call on God first. In those first seconds—tight chest, shallow breath, full-blown nervous system activation—I was relying on myself, planning the escape, and assessing the threat. But when I realized there was no way out, with the patient's eyes fixated on me and the door sealed, prayer became the only exit. In that moment, I prayed not with eloquence or Scripture, but with pure desperation. There were no verses, no filters—just a terrified whisper that said, "God, please," and He heard me. That door opened, that stranger stepped in, and that moment passed.

God doesn't need your polished prayer in times of high need. He wants your whisper and your trembling heart. He wants your simple, childlike trust, even if you don't say it out loud.

I've held onto these verses ever since that day:

Psalm 56:3: *"When I am afraid, I put my trust in you."*

Psalm 23:4: *"Even though I walk through the valley of the shadow of death, I will fear no evil, for you are with me" (ESV).*

Fear will come. But so will God. And if He doesn't calm the surrounding storm, He will steady something inside you. He will send help so you can confidently put all your trust in Him.

Unscript Yourself Toolkit

Permission to Heal

Take one slow breath. If recalling a moment feels unsafe, then choose a lighter prompt or stop. One true line per prompt is better than ten perfect ones.

1) When fear flooded your body.

If it's safe to recall, name a single moment when your body said, "This is not safe" while you were at work. Don't linger on details; focus on what you need.

- What did your body feel first? What boundary or support would have helped you in that exact minute?
- Sentence starters:
  - *"I noticed my ______ tighten / race when ______."*
  - *"The first thing I needed was ______ (time, backup, a closed door, water, to log it)."*
  - *"A boundary that would protect me next time is ______."*

____

____

____

2) When power dynamics muted your voice.

Recall a time a prescriber's status made you shrink, though your clinical judgment had concerns.

- What story about authority was running in your head? What truth about your scope and duty do you want to stand in instead?
- Sentence starters:
  - *"The thought that kept me quiet was ______."*
  - *"The truth I can stand in is that my role includes ______ (final check, dose safety, advocacy)."*

Unscripted Permission Slips:

- You have permission to step away for a few minutes after an episode of aggression: to breathe, reset, and log the incident.
- You have permission to cry and still be a professional. Humanity is not a breach of standards.
- You have permission to believe you are more than the script; you are an advocate, a clinician, and a healer whose voice prevents harm.

Unscripted Affirmation

I am not broken. My presence, judgment, and voice are safety devices worthy of time, respect, and protection, and I'm allowed to heal from what I've carried.

CHAPTER 10

You Are Called to Service Beyond the Script

Intuition goes before you, showing you the way. Emotion follows behind, to let you know when you go astray. Listen to your intuition. It is your spiritual GPS guiding you toward your true destiny.

—Anthon St.Maarten

It was on March 15, 2019, around 1:30 p.m., when New Zealand saw its darkest day. A gunman opened fire on Muslims praying their Friday prayers in a mosque, ending the lives of fifty people in exactly twenty-one minutes.

It had gone deadly quiet in the complex. You could've dropped a pin on the concrete and heard it echo for miles. Then I heard hurried footsteps.

"Did you hear what happened?" the receptionist asked from the doctor's office.

"No, what happened?"

"A maniac has opened fire on people at a mosque. It's live on Facebook."

Surely, this can't be happening. I mean, heck, this is New Zealand, and we're in Christchurch, one of the safest cities. I opened the browser, and the headlines swallowed the screen.

"LOCKDOWN DECLARED IN CHRISTCHURCH"

Then came the line that he would be targeting schools. *Oh my gosh! The kids!* I shrieked, pacing while ringing my husband. "It's okay. I'm going to school. I'll get to them, no matter what," he asserted. I couldn't leave the pharmacy until seven p.m., and the kids didn't return from school until 8.30 p.m. The whole city was immobilized.

As the news disclosed the names of the Shuhada (the martyrs who died), I started tearing up. Some of them were my patients, as I worked in an area with a large migrant community. I knew many of them and their families. They came to me because I spoke their language and understood their culture.

The next day, I called my connections at the local council and offered help, support, translation, and whatever else they needed because I knew some families couldn't speak English. The heartache was beyond comprehension, as innocent lives vanished in the name of hate.

A month later, I received a call—the kind you don't expect when you first step into pharmacy, when your world feels limited to dispensary counters and endless scripts. I was appointed to the Ministerial Advisory Group within the Department of the Prime Minister and Cabinet. A group entrusted with advising on the government's response to the Royal Inquiry into the Christchurch mosque attacks. The goal was to help shape policies and initiatives to ensure safety measures are implemented post-attacks and into the future to maintain social cohesion and community well-being.

Not only was I humbled to work so closely with the Prime Minister and cabinet ministers, but I was honored to serve people who had lost so much. It was the least I could do—to use my governance, advocacy, and health knowledge to fight for the rights of people whose grief I could feel in my bones. It wasn't just an obligation; it was a moral duty. As someone who understood not only their language and culture but also their challenges, their healthcare barriers, and their trauma, I carried that weight differently. It was sobering, sacred work.

And maybe that's what I want you to take away from this experience.

Sometimes the doors that open aren't the ones you would ever script for yourself, but they reveal that the skills you've honed in silence and service have prepared you for conversations you never imagined being invited into.

It was a role my degree hadn't prepared me for, but God saw in me what I couldn't see in myself; He opened the door and said, "Walk through." Some roles require credentials and tidy checkboxes, while others call you to a different kind of service beyond the script. Yet we so often see ourselves as far more unqualified than we really are. But what if, instead of planning your career step by step, you embraced the willingness to evolve, to serve and support beyond the title? To step up and purposefully lean into opportunity within and outside the pharmacy. To follow the Unscripted path you are destined for.

Unscript Yourself Echoes

Before I take you further on this journey, let me pause and ask you a question:

What pain have you witnessed that you haven't yet translated into advocacy?

Every day, in countless ways throughout our practice, we witness suffering in all its shapes and forms. And as much as it aches, that pain can be turned into service. For me, that contribution took the form of advocacy. I've walked through enough pain and adversity to know what it feels like to be shattered. We've all endured something, whether it's bullying, burnout, illness, job loss, or grief. But have you ever thought of turning that experience into a way to contribute and help others?

Though some experiences may feel like punishment, they are there to help you evolve. I wouldn't have thought in a million years that a pharmacist who once made mistakes that could have cost lives would one day be appointed to the very committees that protect them.

That's why I say that a pharmacist's role extends far beyond the four walls that confine us. We already know how to advocate for safe medication use. So how can we use that same voice to advocate for our communities? How can you show your community that you are a human and a professional, that you care and can contribute to their well-being in all its facets? We belong at the table where decisions are made because we carry the stories, the suffering, the insights, and the cultural fluency to bridge the gaps.

This is what I call the deepening of the pharmacist's identity. So this is your permission to show up fully, not just behind the counter, but in councils, on boards, and in political rooms. Because you are not only a clinician; you are a cultural translator, an advocate, and a first responder to humanity.

Somehow, in between ministerial briefings, pharmacy council reports, and a body slowly slipping into rebellion, I won double awards at the New Zealand Primary Healthcare Awards 2020 when I was barely holding myself together. It's that slip that happens when you decide to be everything to everyone while offering nothing to yourself.

Some days, while dispensing, I noticed patterns, like when you question why you're dispensing a copious amount of a particular drug. One pattern I noticed while dispensing was the amount of paracetamol being handed out—boxes of it. It transpired that we had several patients with osteoarthritis (OA) in our community. Around that time, I had just completed my CPD on osteoarthritis treatment, and I knew what the latest research was saying: acetaminophen (paracetamol), despite being the go-to intervention, was not effective at improving pain or function in OA patients. Exercise and manual stretch therapy were far more beneficial. So I partnered with local physiotherapists to create the Osteoarthritis Mobility Project—a research-informed, exercise-first, workshop-delivered program designed to educate, strengthen, and restore movement to patients living with OA.

The program won the Research and Education Award in the 2020 New Zealand Primary Healthcare Awards, alongside the Community Pharmacy of the Year Award, for exceptional service, interprofessional collaboration, and tailoring our services to the needs of our community.

You'd think that would've felt like enough. Those awards were an honor; don't get me wrong; I poured my heart into that work. But standing on that stage, smiling for photos, and shaking hands with decision-makers left me with a strange sense of detachment. While I was being praised as a leader, a change-maker, and a role model in pharmacy, I was also quietly burning out under the load I was carrying alone. If you've ever been celebrated while secretly drowning, you're not alone.

That's the strange thing about recognition: it doesn't always land where you think it will because your soul knows the difference between being recognized for your work and the burden it costs to do that work.

But the real win was seeing patients move differently and live differently. Those awards taught me that a pharmacist's potential is limitless, that you can do things the system never trained you to do. Your only real limitation is the script you believe about what's possible. Find a problem. Be the solution. Show the impact. Work alongside others who share your vision, and the recognition will follow, whether publicly or in the quiet shift you make in your patients' lives. But I assure you, it will follow.

Your only real limitation is the script you believe about what's possible.

Operating without a technician for many days, dispensing and checking after myself while simultaneously providing all the other services pharmacists were expected to deliver (counseling, vaccinations, chasing doctors, reassuring patients, apologizing for delays) exhausted me to my bones. My excitement for what I once considered purposeful work slipped through the cracks of the dispensary, and the mundaneness of life behind the counter numbed me. It showed up in a silent, creeping grief—the kind that doesn't make a sound but eats away at your energy and your nervous system.

Then came COVID-19—the dreaded pandemic that brought out the best and the worst in pharmacists. I believe this was the most profound time in the history of pharmacy. We stood together, united across the globe. We vaccinated. We prescribed Paxlovid. And we remained open when all other healthcare avenues were closed. I've always admired how pharmacists step up in every opportunity to shine their clinical light, especially when it came to overcoming the complexities of prescribing Paxlovid. That was a time when I truly appreciated being a pharmacist.

Like many pharmacists, my exhaustion levels skyrocketed. Eventually, that slow-drip unraveling culminated in something my body could no longer ignore—stress, illness, exhaustion—and it all came to a head during the height of the pandemic, in the middle of a lockdown. I remember everything going black. My heart raced like a stampede of horses as sweat soaked through my uniform. My hands trembled so violently that I couldn't hold a pen. I somehow made it to the pharmacy doors, pulled them down with what little strength I had left, and called the pharmacy owner: "You need to come immediately. I feel so faint."

She arrived in minutes. The medical center next door refused to come near me, assuming I had COVID-19. A few minutes later, I was admitted to ED, my heart rate at 150 bpm, temperature over 105.8°F (41°C), drifting in and out of focus, asserting to everyone who would listen that this wasn't COVID-19, but they still placed me in isolation anyway. They kept me there and poked, tested, and speculated until, a few hours later, the diagnosis changed: septic shock, secondary to pyelonephritis—a life-threatening kidney infection. I was admitted to the ICU, and after arguing through a half-conscious fog, I resisted the PICC line until I could no longer refuse it. A PICC line (peripherally inserted central catheter) is a long, thin tube threaded from a vein in the arm to one near the heart. It's used for extended IV treatments, but it carries risks such as infection, clots, and bleeding. I didn't fully grasp what it was, despite being a pharmacist. I knew it sounded invasive and was dangerously close to my heart. *It's wild how quickly your medical knowledge disappears when you're the one in the hospital gown.*

I was there for a few days, where time lost all meaning, and all I could hear was the hum of machines, the shuffle of nurses, the beeping of monitors, and my own stubborn heart trying to claw its way out of that sterile place. I hate hospitals. I think I drove every nurse and doctor mad with my constant pleading to go home. Eventually, they agreed. Still covered in wires and cannulas, I was discharged to self-administer intravenous antibiotics via a PICC line from home. "We have never done this before," they said hesitantly, unsure if they were allowed. "I'm a vaccinating pharmacist. I'll take full responsibility. I know what I'm doing, and I can't stay here another day."

They referred me to specialist nurses to train me to flush the line, unclog it, and administer IV antibiotics at home. I went back home to finally "enjoy" lockdown with my family, whom I hadn't seen for over two weeks because visitations were prohibited then. That was the most isolating experience of my life, both physically and emotionally. Lying there in an uncomfortable hospital bed, trapped in an under-resourced ward where it seemed to take forever for anyone to come when I needed help, I remember thinking, *How does anyone recover in a place like this?* I saw how broken the system is when the caregivers are stretched so thin that compassion becomes a luxury, rationed like medicine itself.

The excruciating pain of kidney stones compounded that experience, and the medical staff gave me what felt like bucketloads of opioids, none of which seemed to touch the pain. When I expressed that I was still in pain, I was met with that look—that subtle, crushing, silent look that says, *You're exaggerating and being difficult. Maybe you're drug-seeking.* Those suspicious looks only compounded the pain.

That exact experience is what led me down the path of pharmacogenomics. I never learned about it from an article or a conference. It was my own mismanaged health experience, and being numbed into silence, that revealed what was missing in healthcare. When the medications didn't work, when the pain didn't subside, when the doses piled up, and the side effects mounted without relief, I started searching for answers. The medications weren't broken, and I wasn't either. It was that a match had never existed in the first place. Four months later, a pharmacogenomic test confirmed what I already felt deep down: my genetics are the problem.

I eventually recovered; thank God for IV antibiotics. But I left that health experience with one fundamental lesson: This is what happens when you chronically deprioritize your well-being. I had a urinary tract infection for over two weeks, and I dismissed it with over-the-counter medicines—not because I didn't know better, but because I didn't dare to ask for sick leave. These are the times when your inner perfectionist

► **PRO-TIP**

In case you didn't know: Pharmacogenomics (PGx) is the science of how your genes influence your response to medications. It helps explain why some treatments work for one person but cause side effects, or no effect, for another. Think of it as a clinical compass. It's not about replacing guidelines but using them more precisely.

pharmacist worries too much about the chaos of being absent; you care too much for your patients, and in the process, you neglect your well-being.

I worked myself to the bone. It was a constant state of apathy and over-caring, a painful contradiction. What I had lost was my alignment. Only later, in those quiet moments of self-reflection that happen years later, did I learn that recognition without alignment still hollows you out. Burnout isn't necessarily about working long hours but about the misalignment between what you want to do and what you are actually doing. I could no longer work as the only pharmacist, forty-five hours a week while raising kids, or barely make real patient contact because I was stretched too thin. That constant, unrelenting internal dialogue killed me slowly.

My brain was saying, *Are you crazy? You can't resign again. What will people think?* My body was saying, *Umm, you nearly died. You can't keep operating this way. You can't handle this chronic state of working understaffed.* My spirit and intuition whispered, *You know there is more for you to tap into. But you can't tap into it while you're bound here. Your health experience was your awakening. You can always come back to this if you fail.*

With all that inner turmoil swirling, I was up all night, secretly typing out my resignation letter, too afraid that someone might talk me out of what my mind and body desperately wanted. I told myself I'd sit on it for exactly twelve hours—*one more working day*—and if I returned with the same emotions, I would hand it in.

The pharmacy owner came in for her weekly lunchtime visit the next day. She did her usual check-in, asking how things were going, and I replied with one-word answers because I couldn't fake being okay anymore. The words came out of my mouth before my brain had the chance to filter them: "I can't do this anymore. I can't keep working alone with no help. I almost died of burnout. I'm resigning."

I think she was expecting it. She didn't appear shocked but gave me a soft, almost knowing look, as if to say, "*I understand.*" Then she asked, "What's next?" And I replied with an honesty that didn't scare me anymore, "I dunno. Certainly a break. And maybe I will find a way to work that doesn't burn me out."

And so I resigned, not dramatically and not after months of planning or mapping out my next move, but in a calm, rational moment of clarity I'd never felt before. One decision, in one courageous moment, with no plan for the future and no roadmap. Only an overwhelming sense, right there and then, a voice inside that said, *You can't keep going anymore. Something has to shift.* That's often when change happens, as Tony Robbins, a well-known motivational speaker, says, "When the pain of staying the same is greater than the pain of change."

It was scary as heck because stability is sacred in my family, and I knew what it would look like to them. I knew the stares I would get—the questions and the guilt that would follow. And yes, they all came. Yet again, my family looked at me as if I were an ungrateful twit. *"Why on earth would you leave a good-paying, stable job without any plan forward?"* they asked over and over. I didn't have an answer that would make sense to them. Deep down, I knew that life had something better for me, something that aligned with who I was becoming. That whisper inside me—my intuition that had been trying to get my attention for so long—had never failed me before. And so I followed it. I took the risk. I bet on myself. Even with everything I've had to navigate and all the challenges that came with stepping into uncharted waters, I can honestly say I've never regretted my decision. Not once.

I continued the path that was *Unscripted On Purpose*—a path that was mapped not by certainty, but by conviction. A path that doesn't promise ease or clarity but feels like liberty, like truth. I stepped out of that era with one vow: *No more living on autopilot. No more dissonance. From this point forward, I will listen to my intuition and choose alignment and meaning.*

Unscript Yourself Echoes

You can't fix yourself while staying bound to what's breaking you.

I say this with the deepest sense of understanding, infused with urgency: *You can't design a future while clinging to the past.* The two cannot coexist.

You can't become the next version of you while holding onto the past version of you. Equally, you can't fix yourself while remaining bound to the exact thing that is breaking you. It's like trying to glue together a piece of chinaware you hold dear, only to drop it on the floor every time you mend it, shattering it into more pieces again and again until the shards turn to dust. Until there's nothing left to piece back together into any reasonable shape or form.

Similarly, you can't grow in the same environment that keeps depleting you. You either fix the environment or fix the story you're telling yourself about why you have to stay. And yes, I tried to change my mindset. I really did. But eventually, my body gave in because I was carrying too much disappointment, too much work, and too much misalignment for any mindset shift to hold, which manifested as burnout.

Burnout isn't about long hours. It's about soul misalignment. It's what happens when you betray your calling slowly until your body forces you to listen. It's when you choose politeness over conviction. Fixing what is broken in you requires commitment and conviction. A vow to choose alignment, meaning, and purpose every single time. And you'll know when you've found them because you'll feel them first in your body long before your brain has any language for it. You'll hear your soul say, *This feels like me. This feels right deep down.* Even when the whole world is against you. That is what *Unscripted On Purpose* feels like.

Faith Echoes

Stop seeking all the answers. Trust the process, the calling, and, most of all, trust God.

Sometimes God doesn't give you the whole map. He gives you only *a whisper*, a gentle nudge that appears in the form of an experience or words someone speaks to you. You know those moments when you *feel Him*, and you *know* it's Him. That's His way of calling you toward the dream He has already imagined for you.

This dream, frustratingly, doesn't come with a five-year plan or a guaranteed outcome, only with a knowing in your spirit that who you are no longer serves who He created you to be.

Deep down, I was staying in that job out of fear—fear of failure, of being judged, of walking away from a job so many others would kill for. But God calls us to walk by faith, not by sight, and not by the script. Though it is important to have a contingency plan, which, in my case, was another round of job applications, but this time I had a better CV, and that gave me enough reassurance to forge ahead, Unscripted.

There's a verse that carried me through that time:

Isaiah 30:21: *"Whether you turn to the right or to the left, your ears will hear a voice behind you, saying, "This is the way; walk in it."*

That voice might not shout, but it will never lead you astray. Even when the path is Unscripted, He walks it with you. I chose the only path that felt true—the one that was *Unscripted On Purpose*, lit not by logic or guarantee but by the quiet knowing that God doesn't always show you the whole road, only the next right step. And for me, the next right step with Him beside me was better than walking alone, misaligned, stumbling, falling, and eventually breaking.

Unscript Yourself Toolkit

Permission to Serve Beyond the Script Without Losing Yourself

Bring your honest self. Forget tidy answers. One messy truth is worth more than polished silence.

What is one way you could serve your community beyond the script? Recall one moment of pain you've witnessed that could be turned into advocacy.

____

____

____

Where are you applauded but misaligned, and what single boundary would bring you back to yourself?

____

____

____

If you are feeling misaligned in your current role and you gave yourself twelve hours to tell the truth, what would your resignation letter say? (And what contingency plan would you have?)

____

____

____

BONUS Journaling Prompt:

Write a conversation between your brain, your body, and your spirit. What are they each saying about your current work or life season? Whose message is the loudest? Who is being silenced?

Unscripted Permission Slips

- You have permission to carry grief into action, not just into silence.
- You have permission to serve beyond your title, even when the

system doesn't invite you.

- You have permission to leave what breaks you, even without a five-year plan, and choose alignment instead.

Unscripted Affirmation

I will no longer bind myself to what breaks me. I will choose alignment, meaning, and purpose every single time because I am called to service beyond the script.

Unscripted Tips

#1: From Idea → Impact (in five steps)

This is my framework for implementing successful projects in healthcare:

1. **Spot the pattern**: Identify one recurring pain point (e.g., paracetamol overuse in OA).
2. **Scan the evidence**: Review guideline summaries and statistics.
3. **Partner up if appropriate**: Look for one allied clinic (e.g., physio or GP).
4. **Pilot and measure**: Choose three metrics (before/after pain score, step count, medication use).
5. **Show the impact**: Create a one-pager and share it with funders and associations.

#2: Recognizing Burnout Beyond "Tired."

I've added this tip because it is what I wish I had known. We all blaze in silence, and I want pharmacists not just to survive, but to thrive. Burnout in pharmacists doesn't always show up the way we expect. It's not only fatigue or irritability; it's often masked behind over-functioning and robotic compassion, and it goes beyond merely dreading Mondays or blaming the workload.

Here are some signs that you may be quietly burning out, even if you're still performing:

- You feel detached from patients you once cared deeply for.
- You've experienced physical symptoms (fatigue, headaches, insomnia, infections) that you keep dismissing.
- Your empathy is replaced by numbness, frustration, or guilt.
- You fantasize about quitting but immediately shame yourself for the thought.
- You catch yourself repeatedly saying, "I should be grateful, but I'm not."

Burnout isn't a weakness; it's a signal. Ignoring it doesn't build resilience; it erodes purpose. If your work is costing you your health, clarity, and sense of self, then it's time to pay attention.

PART V

The Becoming

"If you don't build your dream,
someone else will hire you to help build theirs."

—TONY A. GASKINS

CHAPTER 11

You Are Called to Conviction, Not Credentials

Don't downgrade your dreams just to fit your reality. Upgrade your conviction to match your destiny.

—Stuart Scott

I couldn't sit with the guilt of leaving mid-pandemic, so I left shortly after the worst of it had passed. I felt a mixture of happiness and loss. It was a feeling of finally having some agency, though I had no idea what on earth I was doing. I didn't have another job lined up, nor a version of myself waiting in the wings. I had only fatigue in my bones and a hundred questions running through my mind that all began with, *What now?*

My last day as a community pharmacist felt like standing at the edge of a cliff. Patients came with flowers, chocolates, and cards that said things like, "Thank you for always caring," and "You are the only one who ever explained things to me." There were hugs I didn't know how to receive and tears I didn't feel I'd earned. I smiled because that's what you do. I said goodbye, though part of me was still clinging to the edge of the dispensary bench, hoping someone would talk me out of it. These are the moments when your brain aches from the inner battle and confusion. But somewhere in the ache, beneath all the exhaustion and unmet potential, is a whisper you can't ignore. I felt an unmistakable sense and presence of a Call to More. I just didn't know what it looked like.

As soon as I walked out the door for the last time, my mind whispered, *Did I do the right thing? Am I a coward for walking away?* But my health was shattered, and all I could see was the exit sign. Sometimes the only catalyst to make things work out is to have your back to the wall because your life depends on it. The fear of failing not only those who are watching you closely but also yourself can be your biggest motivation to keep striving forward.

It was around that time that I started writing online. Somewhere between burnout and "What's next?" was a blank space that writing filled. It was just scribbles in an online blog made up of loose sentences—quiet reflections on the lessons the pandemic had wrung out of us—the kind that I can't read now without cringing. I published it on LinkedIn. It wasn't polished, but it was honest. To my surprise, it struck a chord with people, so I wondered if it should see the light of day and live beyond a feed in an app. Suppose it might find a home in our national pharmacy magazine. I stopped wondering and sent it to the magazine's editor with zero expectations. That email became the start of my publishing journey.

I'll forever be grateful to the Pharmacy Today editor, Ruth Brown, for being the first person in the professional world to look at my writing and say, "This is worth publishing." Writing has been my therapy ever since. It has shaped me in ways I never predicted. It sharpened my thinking and fed a part of my creativity I didn't know was hungry, making me a better problem-solver and a more honest version of myself. I never imagined I'd be a writer, not with English as my third language. But you don't know what you're capable of until you try, until you lean into curiosity. And trying, I've learned, means accepting that rejection is a possibility. It's the reason I've knocked on so many doors, pitched ideas I wasn't sure I was ready for, and sent messages to inboxes I never thought would be read. Rejection is the only door to acceptance.

Rejection is the only door to acceptance.

Unfortunately, bills don't pause when your body does. I gave myself a couple of weeks to breathe and plan. Locuming felt like the most flexible option since I wasn't tied to a permanent contract. I even wondered if all I needed was a new place to reset. So I posted in our pharmacist locum Facebook group, and within minutes, the messages rolled in. And somehow, of all places, I ended up back at the pharmacy where I'd done my internship year. Full circle or foolish? I still haven't decided.

The owner, my former preceptor, asked me to cover his absence for two weeks. He trusted me to hold the fort, and part of me still felt I owed him something, especially after the way I'd left. So, I agreed to work for two weeks. But the moment I walked through those doors, my body gave me its own answer. I had flashbacks of the errors I'd made in that space—mistakes I'd carried like scars I couldn't explain to anyone. Just looking at the packing corner gave me goosebumps. The air felt heavier than I remembered, and so did I—not with shame but with the weight of everything I'd survived since. And that's when it became clear: this wasn't about needing a new workplace. I needed to be released. I needed to get out of community pharmacy, at least for some time, because of what I'd endured inside it. I needed to escape from the bullying, the harassment, and the trauma that had slowly seeped into my nervous system over twelve years.

It was also around that time that COVID-19 vaccination centers urgently needed staff for administering vaccinations. So, after finishing that locum stint, I was summoned to help out. I had hoped that a minor task might give me the ease I needed to recalibrate my system. But three weeks in, I knew it wasn't my lane. The work mattered, but it simply didn't ask for the kind of clinical problem-solving I'm wired for. We are trained to think, counsel, and connect—to ask why a patient isn't adherent, to untangle confusion, reduce harm, and optimize therapy. But I felt like I was narrowing my scope to a single function while preventable medicine-related harm persisted.

I had no choice but to forge a path. It was becoming painfully clear that I had too many ideas that refused to stay quiet, too much confidence that made the room uneasy, and too many convictions I could no longer swallow for the sake of keeping things smooth. I still cared deeply about my career, but I also saw the pain of every pharmacist trying to challenge the system, and I couldn't keep pretending I didn't feel it too.

I had evidence of being a problem-solver; the awards cracked something open. I caught a glimpse of what might be possible if I stopped waiting for permission and let myself be led by conviction. And if no one were willing to open the door for me, then I'd build a door myself.

Around that time, I came across a digitally led healthcare provider launching in New Zealand while scrolling through LinkedIn, and something inside me stirred. I remember thinking how incredible it would be if they had a pharmacist embedded in their team—someone offering remote, pharmacist-led services and patient care that wasn't confined by counters or consult rooms.

The idea felt less like a thought and more like a sense of alignment tugging me toward uncharted territory. I typed the message, then hesitated. I told myself, *Katrina, what on earth are you doing messaging a CEO directly?* But another voice—quieter and stronger—whispered, *What's the worst that could happen? Rejection? You've survived that.* So, without thinking, I reached out to explore adding a pharmacist to his team. I was flabbergasted by the response, *"Love your background. You're a go-getter. Congratulations on all your awards."*

He scheduled a fifteen-minute virtual meeting for me to make a case for why a pharmacist might belong on a team of virtual doctors and nurses. To offer a pitch that would either open a door or close it. To articulate something that had been burning in my chest for years—a reimagining of what pharmacy could look like beyond the counter.

It was in preparing for that pitch that I learned the art of negotiation—the profound shift of learning to make my case not by listing credentials, but by painting a picture of what was possible. That shift lay in changing my mindset from "What's in it for me?" to "What's in it for them?" After our conversation, he invited me to present my ideas in person to his leadership team. I was nervous, but I had already made a quiet vow to myself: *I would no longer shy away from unknown rooms or uncharted ideas, especially the ones that felt bigger than me.* I finally knew that growth begins where comfort ends.

I created a pitch deck that reflected what I'd always known in

► **REFLECTION**

What idea do you need to stop asking permission for? No one will give it to you because you've owned it all along.

my bones: pharmacists add value to medical teams not only as dispensers but also as medicine-optimization experts. I had the most unnerving flight of my life while traveling, rehearsing the presentation in my head with every cloud I passed through. I spoke about the impact of nonadherence, the burden of preventable admissions, and the ripple effect of medicines optimization. I backed it up with data, evidence, and everything I could find that might make them pause and consider the need for a pharmacist on their team.

They offered me the role on the spot, then asked me to choose my hourly rate and write my job description to shape what this role could become for myself and future pharmacists they hire. And it all started in a moment of embracing curiosity and conviction in the path I chose, despite the uncertainty.

I began by focusing on what would ease pressure on doctors and nurses—answering medication-related queries, providing rapid clinical input, and serving as the first point of contact for anything medicine-related. I layered in clinical audits, medication reconciliation during transitions of care, and medication reviews where gaps and risks were hiding in plain sight. But the greatest challenge wasn't the work; it was the invisibility. It was gently and consistently helping doctors get used to the idea that there was now a pharmacist in the room, someone who could carry a decent chunk of the clinical load. To do that, you have to embed yourself in their rhythm. I attended every clinical meeting, delivered weekly clinical education sessions, wrote drug bulletins, and summarized updates on reimbursement changes and clinical alerts. In roles like this, I learned you need to do everything under the sun to remind them of your commitment—that you are here for them, that you are trained to help—and slowly, you earn their attention and their trust.

I eventually understood that the tie between pharmacists and doctors needs to be woven through collaboration, mutual understanding, and shared education. Because when they see the difference you can make not only in patient care but also in saving them time, decision fatigue, and cognitive load, you stop being a nice-to-have and become "indispensable."

When they see the difference you can make not only in patient care, but in saving them time, decision fatigue, and cognitive load, you stop being a nice-to-have and become "indispensable.

While building that role, I posted on LinkedIn and shared a glimpse of my career journey. That one small step ended up shaping my career in more ways than I could have ever imagined. Other pharmacists resonated with what I was saying. They reached out with questions, reflections, and requests for advice. Slowly, a community formed, and a following grew. And somehow, from one of the farthest corners of the world, my voice traveled. It taught me something I hadn't learned in any professional development course: in the digital age, careers aren't only built in boardrooms or in silence; they're built through credibility, consistency, and the quiet power of showing up with something true to say that serves beyond yourself.

But that visibility has a price. Some colleagues I once considered peers chose envy over encouragement, filing a complaint that, though baseless, became one of the most confronting seasons of my career. That's when your registration, your livelihood, and your calling are on the line. It humbles you in a way nothing else can. Yet that experience didn't break me. It sharpened me and taught me what no textbook ever could: the price of standing for something is that not everyone will like you. They will come for you with loopholes twisted into weapons and thrown like darts from across the room because you reflect something they don't have: Freedom. Conviction. Alignment. And they'll never say that outright because that would take courage. Instead, they'll mutter things like, "Who does she think she is?" or "She's so full of herself."

And to that, I say yes; I am full of myself, and you should be too. Decide to be full of purpose, full of clarity, and full of the spirit that sustains you. That's when your cup runneth over, and you can give to others. That's when you're able to inspire, uplift, empower, and do the work you were created to do. But don't let the envy or resistance of others dull your spark. Let it sharpen you. Let it refine you. Let it make you strive to reach your Call to More.

If the first lesson I learned was that visibility comes at a cost, the second was that my voice matters. Why? Because it was shaking something loose in people who didn't want to hear it. Their complaints didn't silence me; they empowered me. Their attempts to keep me down only deepened my conviction and solidified my calling.

So if you haven't stepped into that role or launched that idea because you don't feel worthy enough, or because others are doubting you or dimming your light, or because you think another certificate will finally qualify you, I plead with you to stop. You already have what it takes. What's missing isn't proof; it's conviction. It's the courage to decide, to stay the course, and to refuse the complacency of letting society or resistance throw you off. Conviction isn't just about embracing the unknown; it's about saying no to what's quietly undoing you and saying yes to the path that feels true, even when it terrifies you.

Unscript Yourself Echoes

Have you ever found yourself suspended between the illusion of control and the weight of uncertainty, where agency and surrender blur into one?

That space can be the most unsettling of all spaces. It is an internal conflict of you versus everyone else—society, family, and expectations. Yet the internal tug can be so strong that you can't silence it.

That agency you feel is not rebellion; it's relief. It's the moment you listen—to truly attune to your calling. It is not random; it is intentional. And often, it feels like something has finally clicked. It feels right in your bones. It feels like liberation.

That uncertainty, though uncomfortable and even agonizing, can be the thing that propels you forward. It exists to slow you down, to ensure you're not acting from fear or impulse but from discernment. It teaches you to pause before deciding, to move in alignment with that newfound liberation and agency you're reclaiming.

That uncertainty will roar loudest at the beginning of your Unscripted journey because the path is so unfamiliar, and unfamiliarity always stirs up fear. But as you keep walking, that fear softens. Uncertainty becomes less of a threat and more of a companion, reminding you that you're growing.

So if you find yourself sitting in that space—hovering between agency and uncertainty, between control and surrender—rest assured. It means you are on the right path. Don't rush. Take your time, and let it shape you, steady you, and propel you toward living your journey intentionally and on purpose.

Faith Echoes

There are enemies of "the good" everywhere; let them be your fuel for conviction.

There are many good people in this world who will stand alongside you and help you grow. But there are others, for better or worse, who are propelled by envy. It reminds me of Cain and Abel, where envy turned into destruction. That story warns us what happens when envy festers. But for us, the lesson is different: envy can be reframed as fuel, not poison.

Here's how I've learned not to let envy get to me: when I see someone doing something better than I'm able to do, or sitting in a position I hope to reach, I ask myself what they did to get there. I don't resent them; I emulate them, learn from them, and let their story stretch me.

There will always be envious people. Don't let their insecurity become an obstacle to your growth. Let it increase your conviction. Let it be proof that you're on the right path, the one they wish they dared to take. There is room for them, too. But they don't see it that way. Their minds believe in scarcity, that there's only room for one at the top.

When your heart is aligned with His purpose, no matter who stands in your way, God will make a way around them. He doesn't just protect your name; He will repurpose their malice. What they try to bury you with becomes the soil that grows your next chapter, as goes the verse:

Psalm 34:19: *"Many are the afflictions of the righteous, but the Lord delivers him out of them all"* (ESV).

Unscript Yourself Toolkit

Permission to Choose Conviction

Arrive with your whole heart. Let go of getting it "right."
One line of truth can light more than a hundred rehearsed ones.

Can you recall a time when you had to close the door on something misaligned, even when it didn't make sense on paper? Looking back, what did that choice cost you, and what did it set you free to pursue?

____

____

____

Is there an email, pitch, or message you've been wanting to send but haven't because you didn't feel "good enough" or "qualified"? What would your present self, wiser and braver, say to that version of you still hesitating at the cursor?

____

____

____

Where in your life do you need less proof and more conviction? What is one step you can take this week to say no to what's quietly undoing you and yes to the path that feels true, even if it terrifies you?

____

____

____

Unscripted Permission Slips

- You have permission to move forward with conviction alone.
- You have permission to be visible, even if it unsettles others.
- You have permission to press send before you feel "ready" or "qualified."

Unscripted Affirmation

My conviction is my credential. It is enough to carry me into the rooms I once thought were off-limits and to sustain me when resistance tries to throw me off course.

Unscripted Tips:

Success Tips from My Career Chapters

#1: The Brave Send Button

Here is a framework that helps me overcome the hesitation of reaching out to people:

- **Don't wait for perfect.**
  If you wait until your email, CV, or pitch is flawless, the opportunity will pass you by. Conviction beats polish every time.
- **Shrink the risk.**
  Ask yourself: "What is the absolute worst that could happen if I send this?" Usually, the answer is "silence." And silence won't kill you.
- **Reframe rejection.**
  A no isn't the end. It's resistance training. Every unanswered message strengthens the muscle you'll need for the one that says yes.
- **Focus on the "why them?"**
  Don't over-explain why *you* deserve it. Paint a picture of what's in it for *them*, because that's where influence lives.
- **Keep the rhythm.**
  Set yourself a rule: When the cursor hovers too long, hit send. Don't give fear more time to argue its case. I set myself a rule to hit send before fear talks me out of it, and so far, I have no regrets. Press send because your conviction deserves to see the light of day.

#2: The Perfect Pitch:

Pitch with courage, clarity, and conviction, because disruption is often the doorway to progress. This is the framework I use to pitch any idea successfully.

- **Start with their pain.**
  What problems are they carrying that you can solve? Speak their language, not yours.
- **Show the proof.**
  Back up the pain with evidence: data, stories, or patterns that make the problem undeniable.
- **Offer the solution.**
  Frame your idea as the bridge from pain to possibility. Keep it simple, clear, and actionable.
- **Position yourself.**
  Why are you the best one to deliver this? Lean on lived experience, conviction, and results, not just credentials.
- **Spotlight the benefits.**
  Make it clear what's in it for them. Less stress? Cost savings? Better patient outcomes? Spell it out.
- **Demonstrate traction.**
  Show how your approach has worked before or why it will work now. Concrete talk beats hypothetical jargon.
- **Cut the fluff.**
  Be concise, be concrete, be clear. A pitch isn't a novel; it's a mirror that makes them see the problem and you as the solution (or part of it).
- **Dare to disrupt.**
  Don't apologize for your vision. If your idea unsettles the status quo, that's often proof that it matters.
- **Prove sustainability.**
  Growth isn't about a quick win. Show how your solution can endure and scale.

CHAPTER 12

You Are Called to Build

You can build an empire
with the bricks thrown at you.
—David Brinkley

Something had shifted. Though I was working in my virtual pharmacist role, my health issues had shattered the illusion that the system was enough. I couldn't move on and pretend that the experience didn't happen to teach me a lesson.

The answer hit me deep. For the first time, I truly understood what it meant to be trapped in the endless hamster wheel of trial-and-error prescribing, where people question pain, dismiss reactions, and where patients have to earn relief instead of it being a fundamental health right. I thought about how pharmacogenomics could give patients answers before the suffering began, how it could restore trust in the clinical encounter. And I knew that after enduring the pain I did because of a lack of drug response, I would do anything to bring that vision to life.

The science behind it all felt like a foreign language, and I remember feeling completely out of my depth. I was already pursuing a postgraduate degree in clinical pharmacy. On top of that, I had enrolled in a pharmacogenomics certification through a U.S.-based provider. It was chaotic, but somehow, I made it.

► **PRO-TIP**

You don't need a business plan to begin. You need a problem worth solving, and the humility to learn while doing.

I've always believed that knowledge is power, but only if it becomes something more than theory. Only if it turns into impact. Too many pharmacists (including the past version of me) collect credentials like merit badges—proof to the world that we belong in rooms we were already qualified for. Don't get me wrong; they are justified if required for the role you're in, but not as proof of the skills and competencies your degree imparted to you.

I didn't have a business plan. I had a test kit, a handful of questions, and the desire to make sense of it all in the real world. I tested my family first. I never wanted them to go through the string of medical mishaps I did, and, truthfully, I needed guinea pigs!

I wasn't thinking of it as entrepreneurship then. I was thinking about safety—whether this idea actually worked outside a textbook. But later, I realized that what I had done was something far deeper than a gesture of care. It was the first quiet step in building something. I had unknowingly started where so many good things begin: with people you trust, with something that matters before you know what to call it.

While I was still in the early stages of building my side business, the virtual provider I worked for asked me to bring pharmacogenomics in-house into the role I was currently holding. It was equally tempting and validating to know I was building something with such potential. But after a lot of soul-searching (and probably more than a few sleepless nights), I decided to resign—yes, again! But this time, it was different. This time, I had a plan.

I knew that if I stayed to build their business, I'd be killing mine. And there is no pain quite like the pain of burying your dreams while building someone else's. Of depriving yourself of the chance to build something that matters to you. Of walking past the doorway to your legacy until eventually, it disappears. So, if you're standing in that same space, with a half-built dream in one hand and a resignation letter in the other, I see you. I know it's terrifying, but remember that conviction is a safer bet than comfort.

Conviction is a safer bet than comfort.

I didn't have it all figured out, but I had something deeper: an unshakeable trust in the process. I reminded myself that I had built before, that I'd held awards in one hand while quietly doubting myself with the other, and that the depth of my conviction eventually carried me here.

That's the part we forget, isn't it? We talk ourselves into these narratives that we're not ready or not successful enough to do something bold. And yet, if we paused for a moment, we'd see all the evidence that contradicts those beliefs. We forget how far we've come: the jobs we've survived, the pressure we've endured, the way we kept showing up when no one clapped, and the degree that we earned after long years of relentless study. That's the evidence that we are capable of so much more than we think.

For the first time, I had clarity. I was building to give patients answers *before* they suffered, to provide value-based healthcare, and to prove that we don't have to fit the mold to make a difference. Because when your why is crystal clear, your fear will loosen its grip. That's when momentum takes hold.

Though knowing my why didn't send patients my way. That's the limbo no one talks about: when you have an idea, and your heart is ready, yet you don't know where and how to find the people to serve. So I did what I knew how to do: I reached out to clinics, introduced myself, and offered free educational sessions. I explained what pharmacogenomics was, how it could help their patients, and how I could make their lives easier. Some doors closed, and a few opened. It was here that I understood the pressures of start-up life on a microscale. But it was also the space where my old skills came into play. All those moments of pitching, persuading, and building services from scratch had prepared me for this.

As I talked more, my weaknesses surfaced. I wasn't good at selling my skills. So I began consuming every book I could find about persuasive communication and marketing. Not because I wanted to manipulate or sell, but because I was desperate to translate what I knew into something others could understand. If I could rewrite the pharmacy curriculum, I would embed marketing at its core. I would teach the language of impact. We are so often terrible communicators of our own value; we expect others to recognize what we offer without ever naming it ourselves.

The reality is that the kind of learning that rewires you happens only when you start *doing the thing*. My most significant growth came from wandering into worlds far outside the MIMS and the dispensary. I read business books and listened to podcasts on marketing, investing, and politics—topics that had nothing to do with pharmacy. They gave me angles, nuance, and context—tools no textbook ever taught me. I believe that the degree is only the door. The real learning begins when you do what no one taught you. And if all your learning still fits inside a pharmacy curriculum, then you're not growing; you're shrinking.

Providing genuine, value-based care felt like I'd finally found . . . me. I was no longer at the mercy of a payer, nor did I have to work on someone else's terms. Yes, it was hard. There were failures, setbacks, and more stressful moments than I care to count. You're not guaranteed a continuous income stream unless you invest time and energy into visibility and reminding people you exist. When you're employed, that work belongs to someone else, but when you're building something of your own, every part of it belongs to you. And it's those very moments, when nothing is promised and everything feels uncertain, that somehow unearth the version of you that you didn't know you were capable of becoming.

That's when I understood I never fit in because I was willing to take risks to build something that mattered. The voice of intuition became louder than the fear, and silencing it felt far more dangerous than trying and failing. That voice shows up for all of us, and when it does, you can either choose to listen or keep enduring a life that slowly dims your light.

During this time, I began looking outward, curious about what pharmacy looked like beyond our system and what I might learn from those who veered off the default path, especially those practicing in telehealth and pharmacogenomics

► **PRO-TIP**

When you work for yourself, you become your own visibility engine. No one is coming to "discover" you. You must learn to market, educate, and remind people you exist until your value becomes undeniable.

internationally. I connected with others and shared what I was learning: the fears, the flaws, the ideas still half-formed. Along the way, I launched a podcast, and my voice was amplified through the U.S.-based Pharmacy Podcast Network thanks to Todd Eury, carrying it well beyond our shores, until one day I found myself listed in the Top 50 Global Pharmacists—a list I never imagined I'd see my name on. It wasn't because I had the most polished résumé, but because I had spoken aloud what so many were holding in silence. So many of the narratives that keep us stuck aren't personal; they're systemic and global. When you speak them aloud, others feel seen. When you offer a reframe, a solution, a spark, that's when your voice becomes something bigger than opinion. It becomes leadership. Leadership doesn't start with a title; it begins with telling the truth you wish someone else had said.

Leadership doesn't start with a title.
It begins with telling the truth you wish someone else had said.

While I was still building the foundations of my small business, a few pharmacists began reaching out not just to ask about pharmacogenomics but to understand *how* I was doing what I was doing. That's when something clicked. Maybe I had more to offer than patient-facing services.

So I started asking questions: "Would you want to learn this? Would it help?" And I knew that I didn't want to create another CE experience that ticked compliance boxes. I wanted to build something that would give pharmacists the tools to develop independent models of care—something that fused science with strategy. That's when the Australasian Precision Medicine Academy was born.

This was the moment I learned one of the most important truths of my journey: If something is broken, you don't wait for someone else to fix it. You don't wait for permission or precedent. You become the solution that builds what doesn't exist. Take initiative and lead with courage because you know you have it in you.

Yet what no one knows, and what I've never shared publicly, is that I built this business, this program, this version of myself at rock bottom. The irony of it all is that my highest achievement came at the lowest point of my life.

I share this personal moment because, without it, this book would be incomplete. It would show the success without the cost. The foundation of this business was built during a time of personal trauma and rupture so deep that the scaffolding of my life felt like it was collapsing in slow motion, and I was grasping for anything solid to hold. I built this while walking through a divorce I wouldn't wish on anyone, not even my worst enemies.

I recorded modules through tears, in between endless court proceedings that stretched on for months without mercy, inside a two-meter-square room with nothing but a laptop and a sliver of conviction I could barely hold. I did all this while my physical safety was threatened behind the scenes, and I was too afraid to tell anyone how bad things had become. I taught strategies for resilience while still trying to locate my own. I poured out courage while praying not to come undone. And I say this with my whole heart: If I hadn't poured my energy into building, into doing something that challenged me, I don't know if I would've made it through that season. Because if I hadn't been building, I would've been destroying. Slowly… and quietly… I would've destroyed myself.

I share this not for empathy or to make you wince, but to let you know that if you're walking through grief that threatens to undo you, I see you. More so, I want to encourage you. If I could build during such a tough season, then you can too. Because if you wait for perfect circumstances to build something meaningful, you may wait forever. The same ground that nearly broke me became the foundation of an educational program that, against all odds, was later awarded runner-up in the New Zealand Primary Healthcare Awards in 2025. This wasn't a passion project; this was my means of survival, the solid thing I grasped onto when I was falling. This was Unscripting at its finest.

Unscript Yourself Echoes

Have you ever stayed silent through pain and unraveling to protect others?

The worst of all pains is the one that eats away at your soul in silence, over hours, days, and weeks. And you're too scared to share it because sharing it not only breaks you; it breaks those around you who do not wish to see you in pain. Your breakdown would shatter their world. It is then that silence becomes your only escape, when absorbing the pain becomes the remedy.

These are the times we go down one of two routes: either we undergo slow self-destruction because we're holding far more than our emotional bandwidth can handle and internalize those emotions, which manifest as self-doubt, criticism, burnout, and depression. Or, on the rarer path, we use creativity and building as an outlet. This isn't a common route, but any musician or creative will tell you they created some of their best work in their darkest moments.

I know the pain. Too well. The pain of holding it together. The pain of silence. That burden you carry in every moment that you can't share. Of being the mom who does everything, breaking down internally while showing up as a pharmacist. Making those lunch boxes and doing the laundry while facing an internal storm no one sees. Of being that dad who feels like he's carrying the full weight of being the breadwinner, while societal stigma keeps him from ever voicing how heavy it really is. Of being that person in an abusive, difficult, or unraveling relationship, yet turning up with a flawless public façade, masking private despair.

And the pain of turning up to a job that feels like… a job. Nothing but that—a soul-crushing, burnout-inducing role that promises you nothing but a paycheck, which is all society needs from you. Not your talent. Not your potential. Just your compliance. But from that pain, you can and must rise. When you don't know what to do, lean in. Build! Because creating something outside of yourself is often the only way to rise above the circumstances.

This message is for every pharmacist who is building while breaking, teaching while healing, rising while doubting, and silently struggling while their soul is screaming: You are not behind. You are becoming. Start building, even when the bricks are heavy with grief.

I designed the curriculum the way I wished I had been taught. I have sat through enough coma-inducing lectures to know what not to do. So I researched competency-based education until my eyeballs hurt. I fell into rabbit holes about gamification, AI, and student engagement strategies, not because I was an expert, but because I couldn't bear the thought of someone feeling that they paid for an unsatisfactory experience.

I launched messily and asked for feedback, despite fearing the outcome. In the business world, they call it "launching a minimum viable product." It means releasing before you're ready and trusting that refinement will follow. This was hard to fight against my perfectionist tendencies as a pharmacist. What I learned from this initial building phase was that perfect is polished fear.

So I showed up. Over one hundred hours. On camera. I'd tell myself, *Just one module today*, whether I felt inspired or hollow. Some lessons were recorded more than three times because I looked so broken. I had promised something to these pharmacists. Their faith in the idea became my deadline and my reason to press "record" when I wanted to hide.

Eight weeks later, after countless hours of filming in between patient consultations and cold outreach to doctors, I finally launched the beta version. In that moment, two voices collided within me: one, barely a whisper, said, *Well done. You made it despite what you've been through.* And the other (louder and crueler) scoffed back, *Do you really think this is good enough? You've wasted people's money. You've shamed yourself publicly.*

I whispered my lifeline: *God, don't let all this effort amount to nothing.* Then the first response landed in my inbox: *"This is the best educational format I've experienced. Feeling empowered!"* I stared at the words and let them settle into the space where doubt had lived for too long. In that moment, I cried. I could finally exhale for the first time in weeks, and I thanked God for turning the hardship into a harvest and the breaking into building.

I learned that perseverance does pay off, that the universe (for me, that's God) rewards those who refuse to give up on the dream buried deep in their spirit. I've lived it over and over again through every strange detour my career has taken. At every cliff I've stood on, with knees shaking, I still stepped forward. People don't fail because they're not capable; they fail when they don't try.

If I'm being honest, we pharmacists fear risk because it goes against our deeply rooted instincts for vigilance. To check and triple-check, operating with zero risk tolerance, because when it comes to prescriptions, perfection is a nonnegotiable. But that same mindset will kill your creative calling. If you want to choose the path that is *Unscripted On Purpose*, you're going to have to release the rules you were taught and rewrite the ones that serve you now. Because no one is coming to save you!

Every negative experience I endured—every dismissal, every misstep, every time I was overlooked or underpaid—wasn't only for the sake of suffering; it was a wake-up call, a reroute to the Unscripted path. Each one forced me to see that I couldn't sit back and wait for change. I had to *be* the change I was so desperate to see. I had to save myself. I had to stop waiting for the system to reform, for someone to recognize my worth, for a mentor to say, "Now you're ready." I had to become the pharmacist I was born to be—one who lives aligned with her dreams, honors her worth, and serves patients beyond the limitations of the model that boxed her in.

This I know for sure: there is more to every pharmacist than a title. The dream is realized only when you stop shrinking yourself to fit a script that was never yours, when you remember that credentials might unlock the door, but conviction is what builds the room. If I had limited my potential to my degree, I never would've been a writer, an advocate, or a parliamentary advisor. None of the chapters of this book would've been written if I had stayed trapped in the belief that "I'm just a pharmacist."

Once you let go of that belief, growth will follow—I promise you. The most meaningful chapters of your life will begin in the aftermath of fear, in the wreckage of what you believe you need to keep holding on to. Every time I let go of certainty, of safety, of the job I'd built my identity around, I found something more profound. And yes, it cost me. There were days I grieved the titles I left behind. But staying stuck in something that drained me costs more. It cost me joy. It cost my sense of self and agency.

It's wild to think that this once-rejected pharmacist gets to do what I do today: build, teach, write, inspire, host a podcast, lead, and tap into creativity beyond the title. Not because I had a map, but because I followed the nudge, the sacred curiosity—the one that kept whispering, *There's more.* And trust me, it wasn't strategy that got me here. It was God's grace paired with the courage to keep walking forward when I couldn't see what was next.

This isn't the end of the journey but the beginning—the beginning of a career built On Purpose. On connecting with the humans in healthcare, not patients on paper. On remembering that before you are a pharmacist, you are a human. On becoming the best version of yourself, not for promotions or applause, but because you know what's at stake when you don't. On delivering care that goes beyond medication charts and standard protocols. On delivering the *more* you are called to deliver.

You can't find that *more* if you only look through the lens of your title. Because the *more* isn't in identifying as a pharmacist. It's in knowing that you are not just a pharmacist. You are a human beneath the white coat. A creative with a soul. A mum with dreams that don't fit inside a nine-to-five life. A dad with unspoken hopes for his family and long-buried ambitions. A student trying not to lose themselves before the journey has even begun. That's where the "more" is hiding. It's always been there. It was never in the title. It has always been … inside you.

Faith Echoes

Rock bottom isn't punishment; it is preparation.

Rock bottom is hard to describe if you've never been there, and I hope you never have to be. But the closest way I can explain it is this: rock bottom is when you've given up completely, not just on your job but on yourself, your life, on everything.

Rock bottom isn't just depression; it goes beyond that. It's the loss that leaves no light, no door, no breath of relief. Where every path is blocked, every prayer feels unanswered, and it feels like the whole world is conspiring to break you down. And worst of all, you can't find the strength to care anymore.

But through prayer, I came to understand what I couldn't see then: why God allows these seasons. He is not trying to punish you; He is preparing you. He is stripping everything that was built on a shaky foundation. He is cleaning the slate and making space for a new assignment and a renewed mind—for the version of you that can carry the weight of His calling. The one that is aligned with His purpose for your life.

I've had to learn the hard way to trust in God's greater plan for my life. I now understand that loss is sometimes necessary for growth and for stepping into the next chapter God has for me. He can't build a new house on a cracked foundation.

God is not sentimental about seasons. He closes doors not to punish us but to position us. He removes people not to leave us lonely but to lead us into a deeper relationship with Him. And He allows losses not to hurt us but to humble and ready us.

So if you've hit rock bottom or you're carrying burdens from the past, maybe this is your sign to finally put them down, stop asking for closure, and start asking for courage. Stop rehearsing what went wrong and start preparing for what's ahead. Because there is a future you are called to walk into. And you cannot walk freely into it if your hands are full of everything God has already asked you to surrender.

Psalm 126:5: *"Those who sow in tears shall reap with shouts of joy." (ESV).*

Romans 12:2: *"Do not conform to the pattern of this world, but be transformed by the renewing of your mind. Then you will be able to test and approve what God's will is—his good, pleasing and perfect will."*

Unscript Yourself Toolkit

Permission to Build Before It's Perfect

Let go of getting it "right."
One line of truth can light more than a hundred rehearsed ones.

What is one idea you've been sitting on—an idea that perfectionism has kept locked in drafts, notes, or "someday"? What would imperfect execution actually look like?

___

___

___

Think of a time you hit rock bottom. If, alongside the pain, you had given yourself permission to build something small in the middle of it, how might that moment have reshaped your story?

___

___

___

Where is risk calling you right now? What is the one decision you would make if fear of failure or judgment weren't allowed a vote?

___

___

___

Unscripted Permission Slips

- You have permission to start building before you feel ready.
- You have permission to let go of perfectionism and choose progress instead.
- You have permission to see rock bottom not as the end, but as the foundation.

Unscripted Affirmation

I don't need perfect conditions to build. I carry the conviction, the courage, and the first brick already.

CHAPTER 13

Your Call to More Is Unscripted On Purpose

Getting to the More is not a climb, but a homecoming.

—Katrina Azer

This is the chapter I almost didn't write because it felt like I was undoing everything I had written so far. But as the thoughts poured out, I found that, if anything, it completes the book. It is the chapter that comes after you climb the mountain and stand at the top, only to realize that you climbed the wrong mountain.

I built what served patients with heart. I educated pharmacists with soul. I won all the awards I thought would matter. I received external validation—the kind that makes people look twice when they see your bio. And though it felt good, it wasn't enough to silence the ache or fill the space inside me that whispered, *Is this it?* It didn't feel true to my calling. This internal unraveling is what led me to write this chapter.

For years, I intentionally took the Unscripted path by leaning into opportunities that came my way. It was momentum disguised as purpose. And as I continued my pursuit of building behind the scenes, completing projects, collaborating, and chasing external validation, the scaffolding suddenly collapsed. Collaborations crumbled. People walked away. God didn't only close the doors; they slammed shut with a finality I couldn't ignore. And it felt like He was saying: *Stop trying to move forward in the wrong direction.*

I felt broken. And while my business was flourishing, watching these projects fall apart felt like a rejection that pierced me. For too long, I had relied on society to prove my worth. So when doors slammed, I lost my identity. I struggled to express my feelings, so I began to write to cope. I wanted to be an active participant in my unraveling. I wanted to answer the questions: *Is this my life purpose? Is this my calling? Do I have the right definition of success?* I searched. I asked God to help me find His purpose in my life, not the version I crafted out of ambition and the need for validation, but the version He meant for me.

I deliberately put a pause on everything, including my business, which was at its peak performance, and turned away clients. Because if money was meant to fill the gap, it didn't; so it couldn't be the answer. It felt like my accomplishments no longer mattered, and that scared me. If my achievements stopped satisfying me, then what was the *more* I was chasing?

In that pause, it hit me: I was burned out again. But this time, it wasn't because the system was burning me out. This time, I was doing it to myself—gently enough that I didn't notice it. I was trapped in the worldly hustle and grind of chasing metrics and money—the "Look at me! I have it all together!" culture—while I knew full well I didn't. I had wounds from my past, and instead of giving myself grace and understanding to heal them, I chose to stay distracted and busy to forget them. But that came around to bite me. Because that's what happens when you put a Band-Aid on an unclean wound: it doesn't heal; it festers. And that wound quietly deepens over the years, becoming a silent infection you don't realize is killing you.

I needed a reset, so I took a six-month career break, during which I wrote this book. I gave myself permission to search, explore, and find alignment. I knew too well what burnout costs, and if the first time it took away my physical

► **REFLECTION**

Burnout doesn't always come from the system. Sometimes it comes from the stories we tell ourselves about what makes us valuable.

health, this time it was stripping me of my purpose.

I felt the calling deep in my bones to share the load with others. So, I shifted the narrative. I stopped talking about credentials, projects, and strategy, and started talking about the human in me. The tired one who needed healing. The one who still believed there was purpose buried somewhere beneath the protocols. Pharmacists responded to me in emails and DMs, and every response said the same thing: "We are aching too." And in that ache, I saw a mirror. I saw the profession I love cracked open, crying out for something deeper, something real and meaningful. So, I started writing this book.

Writing became my scalpel; each sentence sliced through the scar tissue of old ambition. I wrote everything from the beginning of the journey through to the last chapter (Chapter 12), when I had built my business, gained more recognition, and then paused. It felt—and was—incomplete because I was at the deepest point of my unraveling and didn't have any clarity. The book was about helping you find your Call to More, but I felt like an imposter because I thought I had found mine. But it turns out I hadn't. I paused and prayed: *God, if this is meant to serve people beyond me, then help me complete it.*

I started meditating, exercising until my bones screamed, tapping into hobbies like dancing, skating, hiking, and connecting with God in nature. I volunteered at a local nursing home for seniors. Doing all the things that, for over fifteen years, I considered "not essential" because they didn't make money. They didn't validate me enough.

Slowly, my cup began to fill, awakening a different type of joy. It wasn't the type that lasts for moments. I know too well what that looks like: when you get the award, are happy for a day, then chase the next thing because you feel hollow again. This was the slow-release formulation—the kind that felt truer and more aligned.

If the first round of purposeful Unscripting was all about finding out where I truly fit in society, the second round was all about letting go of it all. To unlearn everything I had come to learn about success and life. I allowed society to shape it and never looked within to shape my own beliefs, and to do the deep work that would break me open and unearth who I truly am beneath the dust that piled over the years. The kind of deep work that requires you to stop running away from hardships, challenging emotions, and scrolling through them aimlessly to numb yourself from the pain of confrontation, instead of feeling your emotions and allowing them to shape you. I found it in pausing and reconnecting with myself again. In sitting with the discomfort of my past, accepting it, and embracing the present. In finding my hobbies and talents. In letting go of everything I've held onto thus far, and redefining what true success means to me.

Amidst that reincarnation, I had a trip booked to the Mediterranean that I planned to cancel because of all the projects that came up. I'd never been big on travel because it didn't feel as validating as the accomplishments of work. But that inner voice said, *You need to go.*

It was the experience I didn't know I so desperately needed. Travel broadens your perspective like nothing else. And it's not only about the food or the places; it's the people, the connection with history, and the richness of different cultures. Travel forced me to find my way back to myself. It touched something so deep within me, a part of me I had never connected with before that was long buried beneath systemic and personal trauma, begging to be healed.

I found that part of me when I watched the sun rise above the Rialto Bridge in Venice, in the colorful doors and draping plants of the white villages in Mykonos. Such extraordinary beauty surrounded me that sometimes it felt unreal. I found beauty in the cobbled streets of Rome, so historic that they gave me goosebumps; it was as if the stones could speak. I found it in the broken columns of the Acropolis that whispered, *Look, I'm broken. But I'm still standing. And you can too.*

I found myself again in simple interactions with strangers: the old, lonely man on the train; the university student who told me about her experience living in a small, isolated town, bringing back so many of my own memories. I found it in the unpolished truth of everything. In the ruins that were left untouched for centuries, portraying the creativity of humans before machines surfaced and took over some of our intellect. We are meant to create, to build, to make what is beautiful, but somehow we have killed that in the name of status and degrees. Perhaps that's the reason for our suffering.

Perhaps the most captivating realization was understanding the power of interdependence in these cultures. Even though they drink, smoke, and indulge—things we often warn patients against—they still live longer, more vibrant lives. Because they thrive on human connection. They don't thrive on independence but on interdependence. On being a cohesive society, not one surviving on the power of individual autonomy—something we miss in our fragmented Western society.

Walking down the rustic white stairs of the Greek villages was soul-awakening. I peered through a door left open and saw a TV with an aerial and a fridge that looked like it was from the eighties. I saw a grandma sitting with her grandchildren on the balcony, hanging washing on the line. They are finding the *more* in looking beyond the material—in simplicity, minimalism and human connection.

It was in those moments that I realized I had been barely existing my entire life and felt more alive than ever. We don't live to work; we work to live. This realization hit deep, and I'm reminded of Bronnie Ware's book, *The Top Five Regrets of the Dying*. She was an Australian palliative care nurse seeking meaning and found it by interviewing people in palliative care. One of the top five regrets of these people is prioritizing work over experiences and relationships. This regret was followed by not living a life true to yourself and pleasing others instead, not investing time in expressing yourself authentically and openly, not maintaining connections with loved ones, and holding on to fear and negativity.[1] All the things that we say we will get around to doing later, as if we can guarantee tomorrow.

I often lost my way, catching the wrong trains and buses and ending up in the wrong villages. Yet in that loss, I found what I had been looking for. When I got lost, I asked people for directions, stopped for a local delicacy, got a cool gift, or saw an ancient ruin that I wouldn't have otherwise seen. In those moments of feeling completely lost, I experienced joy I'd never felt before. I found the real me—the wanderer, the explorer, the one who craves meaning and connection more than material things. But I had lost all of that in my pursuit of external validation.

And it made me question: *What if getting lost means you find your way back to yourself? To your calling?*

We always want certainty before "doing that thing." We want to know whether it will succeed before we proceed. We want every little detail planned for the destination and to know precisely how to get there. But what if the Call to More is found in embracing the spontaneity of life? What if we're brave enough to take that first step with conviction, trusting that the path will unfold? What if we trust ourselves a little more to figure it out, and that real courage lies in accepting the challenge?

And maybe that is the secret of life: to merge with it rather than resist it. To allow it to carry you while you have the best intentions at heart, and to give it back all you could—service, connection, love—a legacy. And take from it what it has to offer—experiences that shape you, enlighten you, and fulfill you. Experiences that help you find your way back to your creative self: the writer, the singer, the artist.

That trip awakened in me the storyteller, the human who thrives on connection and on listening to people's stories. I had been suppressing building relationships and my talents for so long in the name of the chase, but travel helped me reconnect with my true purpose. I found the *more* when I leaned into experiencing life, because that is what life is: an experience. And once I leaned in, I found my true Call to More: *To reach the highest potential that aligns with God's purpose in my life, to embrace every talent I have in His service while helping every human I come across to do the same.*

So, was the climb to the top of the mountain of success fake? No. I served patients, communities, and pharmacists, and it felt fulfilling. But it didn't feel like my calling yet. I thought it was until I was forced to pause, and then I realized that, deep within me, I was doing it for validation more than for purpose. I vowed never to return to my career from a place of seeking validation again, but from a place where my cup is so full, my soul so aligned, that I only take intentional steps to offer service from my heart. What I missed was the intention behind doing the work, which is what I found in the pause.

The Unscripted path of leaning into opportunities will definitely lead to career success, but only when you find your true purpose with intention, and lean into life in a meaningful way. When you get *Unscripted on True Purpose.* Not the "hustle-and-momentum" type of purpose.

The career-success climb can coexist with the calling, but one must lead. If it's your job leading your soul (as in my past), you'll always feel lost. The Call to More lies in being authentic to yourself, in using your talents in service of others for the sake of service, not for validation or reward. Because the pursuit of external validation disguises itself as ambition, and it is exhausting and empty. But the fullness that fills your hollow inside is not found in building a career isolated from your humanity. You have to build the human within you who longs for creativity, meaning, service, and connection. You will find it if you don't confine yourself to a title. You don't have to be either/or; you can be both. A pharmacist and a poet. A clinician and a creator. A professional and a pilgrim. Let that be the rocky foundation you build on, not on the sand defined by others. When you do this, your *more* will reveal itself, I assure you. You were created on purpose, for a purpose, and your calling is grounded in using your talent in service beyond yourself. Your real job is to figure out as soon as possible what that is and honor it. This is what brings true fulfillment.

On our deathbeds, what will matter most is not our bank accounts but the legacy we leave behind. We will not look back and congratulate ourselves on how high we climbed but on how deeply we lived, how heartily we served, how fully we loved, and whether every moment aligned with God's purpose in our lives.

After all the achievements, the successes, the travels, and arriving here, I can tell you this for sure: Finding your Call to More is not a climb but an Unscripted homecoming journey... back to yourself—the human behind the white coat—one who intentionally lives Unscripted and chooses meaning over material, purpose over positions. One who experiences and lives life, not just exists in it. One who chooses internal joy over external approval. One who honors their calling.

Let this be a reckoning to build your life on a robust foundation that is never shaken, and the beginning of your journey to live your life *Unscripted On Purpose.*

This isn't an ending.
This is the part where you lace up your shoes
and start walking in the path that is
Unscripted On Purpose.

PART VI

The Call To More

"There is no greater gift than to honor your calling. It's why you were born. And how you become most truly alive."

—OPRAH WINFREY

CHAPTER 14

The Call to More
What Is It?

The Call to More is not a summons to achievement, but an invitation to become wholly, unapologetically yourself.

—Katrina Azer

I know you've tasted that subtle emptiness—the ache that all the titles, pay raises, or praises of "well done" can't quite fill. Maybe you've wondered, quietly and alone, if you're the only pharmacist who has ever felt this restless, this unfinished, while lying on your bed at the end of a long day, wondering, *Is this all there is to life?*

Maybe you've accomplished more than anyone ever expected of you, yet you still feel hollow inside. Maybe you're so burned out you fantasize about quitting, but you convince yourself to keep going anyway, hoping the next achievement or promotion will finally quiet that ache. The Call to More is that faint pulse that hums, *Is this it,* in the background. It is easy to ignore at first, but eventually it will thunder, and you'll know you can't stay where you are.

In our attempt to correct the emptiness we feel within, we often identify with things (possessions, money, success, status) to fill the ache. And in most cases, despite attaining all those things, we still feel empty. The more you delude yourself into identifying with "things" and force yourself to believe they'll fill that hole, the more miserable you become.

You keep chasing more of the same thing because of one fundamental truth: You are living from a place of lack, of never being "enough" so you continue searching. And searching is a habit that leads to more searching. So you're always looking for the next thing that quiets the ache until eventually, either severe burnout or some tragic life event stops you in your tracks and demands that you reevaluate and realign.

This happens because identifying with things inflates our ego, but it never nourishes our soul. We live in a day and age where the ego is divine and worshiped. Society's version of more is all about the *validation of me.* We never feel enough because we center fulfillment around ourselves and our desires. We become so self-centered. We envy and compare. We become consumed by a finite mindset and lose the abundance life offers. That finiteness leads to a stronger sense of lack, which fuels the need for more, and before you know it, your life evaporates, and you die trapped in the *endless pursuit of more.*

I came across this sobering quote by communication coach Vinh Giang shared in an interview on *The Diary of a CEO*, quoting his father: "A king that knows the limits to his desires will rule a lifetime."[1] The metaphor behind the quote is that kings who conquer more land eventually get killed, whereas the kings who know the limits of their desires rule for a lifetime. In other words, if you continue the outward chase, you'll burn out, but if you look within and lean into the moment and what it offers, you will find peace and contentment in what you've already walked through, survived, built, and become.

The *more* is not a stationary state of being. It is a constant *becoming* of a better, truer, aligned version of yourself. It is letting go of your current identification with material form, dissociating from societal norms, stopping the outward chase, and finding that inward stillness. The Call to More is not answered with material; it is intangible. It is not a summons to achievement but an invitation to become wholly, unapologetically yourself—to live in alignment with your gifts, your purpose, and your deepest joy, not someone else's script.

It's not about denying your ambition but anchoring it. It's about knowing when to stop conquering and start dwelling in your calling, in your truth, and in the blessings already before you. The pursuit of more will not bring you happiness or the joy that surpasses understanding, but living your calling will. Don't be fooled by the tangible things that feel like peace but are only temporary distractions that block true peace.

The *more* you long for is *freedom.* Freedom from everything that keeps you confined—from titles, from the constant chase for money, from schedules. The freedom to just *be.* To be creative, to be more aligned, to be more purposeful, and to pursue meaningful experiences that fill you up.

Your Call to More will be answered when you pause. You will never find it in the hustle of day-to-day life. You're too busy to notice the calling. Pause provides clarity and alignment with what truly matters in your life.

You will find it when you get *Unscripted On True Purpose*—your calling that is waiting for you to tap into. You will find it when you stop being on the receiving end of life and start being on the giving end. When you come from a place of abundance and contribute to the world beyond yourself. When you connect with yourself and have a spiritual practice that gives you faith and hope beyond yourself. When you believe that there is more to your identity beyond your title. As Oprah states, "There is no greater gift you can give or receive than to honor your calling. It's why you were born. And how you become most truly alive."[2]

In the chapters that follow, you'll see that your Call to More is less about what you achieve and more about what you reclaim, reawaken, and finally choose to believe about yourself. It is found in your identity, your purpose, your creative potential, your faith, and your trust in your own intuition.

Let the next few chapters be your permission slip to reclaim your Call to More.

CHAPTER 15

On Identity
Who Are You Beyond "Just a Pharmacist"?

If you don't know who you are beyond the title, it is hard to find your purpose.

—Katrina Azer

How do you define yourself? And who defines who you are? Much of your identity is not defined by you. It's defined by society, systems, expectations, and rarely by who you truly are. Society defines you by what you do, not who you are.

If I asked you to introduce yourself, you'd likely say, "I'm a pharmacist" before you ever said, "I'm a mum," "I'm a dad," "I'm a child of God," or "I'm an artist." We don't name our joy-givers; we name our jobs instead. And though those letters after our names do matter, they trap us when they become the whole story. No wonder we're living in the endless pursuit of more letters and more achievements.

These letters shape not only your identity but also your destiny. Your limitation lies in your identification with your current form, with your title, with the name tag you once proudly wore that now feels more like a leash than a legacy. That's why you end up chasing the wrong *more*—one filled with external validation, not the quiet conviction of becoming your truest self.

Identifying yourself simply as you, not by your position in society, will feel unfamiliar, scary, and even disorienting, as if you've lost your place in the world. But that's where real freedom begins. This is the freedom I talked about in the last chapter—the kind that doesn't come from quitting your job or dropping the title, but from not confusing any of it with who you truly are. Let go of the title and the story you've told yourself about who you have to be based on societal standards. Only then will you find the hidden you—the one with all your talents, ideas, and skills not yet explored—buried beneath the scripts, aching to come alive. The version of you that exists far beyond your imagination.

So who are you? It is the answer to this question that leads to your life's meaning and purpose. Your job may be what you do, but it was never who you are. You are not the script; you are the soul that outgrew it. If your name tag were stripped away, what would be left? What parts of you have gone unnamed for too long? What identities have you hidden because they weren't "serious," "stable," or "approved"?

Your degree was awarded by a university, and your title was handed to you by a company, but your identity is yours to reclaim. It is deeply rooted in your past, your history, your culture, and your faith. If you don't know who you are beyond the title, it is hard to find your purpose.

You were never just a pharmacist. You were always something far more profound. And if no one has ever given you permission to define yourself beyond your role, consider this: You do not need a title to be significant. You need to believe in the truth of who you are. And truth can't be credentialed; it can only be remembered. You are the only one keeping you from the better version of you because your current identity feels familiar; it feels like home, but it is actually binding you.

I am *inviting* you to pause for a few minutes and rewrite the script that has been defining you. You may feel this is a bit woo-woo or that you're short on time, but if you don't reconnect with who you truly are, you will never truly find that alignment and will stay trapped in the pursuit of the more that never fills you.

Work on the following framework. Write it out. Let it evolve if it needs to. But please make space for it. Because everything that comes next—your purpose, your meaning, your *more*—depends on this. This is not just an exercise. This is your *becoming.*

You were never meant to be only what the world could see. Let yourself be named by what grounds you, what fills you, and what you're willing to reclaim. You are the story waiting to be written. Let's reclaim your identity one line, one truth at a time.

The Unscripted Identity Toolkit

Reclaiming Who You Are Beyond the Scripts

We've been told to define ourselves by our titles. But what if we defined ourselves by what grounds us—our roots, faith, and tradition—instead of what boxes us in?

I acknowledge the mental effort it takes to answer this question. You have to sit with yourself for hours, maybe days, to access the deeply rooted identity before it was sugar-coated with society's definitions.

The Unscripted Identity Statement Framework

I am [your name], a creation born of [beliefs, source, or spiritual truth], rooted in [faith or philosophy, if any], descended from [your lineage, cultural heritage, or chosen legacy], and purposed to [your impact, intention, or reason for being].

Example: After a two-day retreat of connecting with God, nature, and myself, here is my version:

[I am Katrina, a Child of God, divinely breathed into being by the Creator, an indigenous Egyptian and descendant of the pharaohs, ancestrally rooted in the Coptic Orthodox Christian faith, and eternally purposed to fulfill God's calling: to help people reach their highest potential and find their purpose in Him.]

Now it's your turn.
Reflection questions to help you:

- *What parts of your identity have gone unnamed, unspoken, or unclaimed?*
- *How much of who you are has been scripted by others?*
- *What would your Unscripted Identity Statement say if no title were required?*

CHAPTER 16

On Purpose & Meaning
Why Are You Here?

What you're craving is the absence of wanting anything. The quiet joy of living—in being fully present and fully enough in the life you already have.

—Katrina Azer

If knowing who you are beyond the title is the foundation, your "why" is the reason you pursue the Call to More. It is what carries you through the fog, the setbacks, and the days when nothing seems to make sense.

If you are still unclear about your identity, maybe you haven't yet met yourself beneath the script. *Who you are* is the *vehicle. Why you are here* is the *destination.* You need clarity on both to drive forward with conviction. Most of us never ask why we're here because we're too busy surviving the script. And if we ever do, the discomfort of the exercise makes us want to look away. But asking is the first step to escaping the cycle of meaninglessness.

Let's get crystal clear on the difference between purpose and meaning.

Purpose is future-focused—the vision or mission that pulls you forward, the answer to "Why am I here?" or "What do I strive to achieve in life?"

Purpose does not come from external achievement or material possessions. It's not tangible. If you tie your purpose to the material, you'll never achieve enough to feel fulfilled.

Meaning is rooted in your past and present. It asks, "What gives my life significance right now? What stories, memories, or choices enrich my existence?" It is your experience of life, your story, and what you choose to do in the present to deepen that story or experience.

If purpose is the destination, meaning is the journey and its richness. Meaning anchors you when your purpose wavers. Meaning is found in choosing the right thing, not the next thing. For me, that looked like turning down more work and chasing more experiences that nurture me. These weren't dramatic moves but small, defiant rebellions against a culture that says we are only as good as what we produce. I ended up feeling richer than I ever had. These moments—sunlight through the leaves, laughter at the dinner table, a plane ticket to somewhere I'd never been—became the quiet architecture of a meaningful life.

Meaning is also found in service—in doing work that transcends your personal success. That helps people with no expectations. And that brings us back to the deepest kind of meaning: we are not here to be impressive. We are here to be of use. Martin Luther King Jr. said it best, "Not everybody can be famous, but everybody can be great, because greatness is determined by service."[1]

Many people say their meaning comes from pursuing something. That's because the state of pursuit is associated with the release of dopamine, and studies have shown that dopamine levels fall just before you get what you want, meaning the chase is more exciting than achieving the end goal. Thus, the journey matters more than the final destination, which is why it is essential to pursue experiences that enrich your life.

But to pursue these experiences, we need time and capacity. So, the essence of your search for *more*, and aligning with purpose and meaning, is having the freedom to choose how you live, not society's pre-approved version of "how you should be living."

Unfortunately, society's definition of living is "buying" the *more* instead of "living" the *more*; that's why you never cease wanting. What you're craving is the *absence of wanting* anything. The quiet joy of living—in being fully present and fully enough in the life you already have.

Hence, the real problem is how to escape the cycle of always wanting.

Escaping the cycle of wanting the fake more and finding real freedom only happens when you are crystal clear on who you are—your identity—and why you are here, which is your purpose and meaning. Then you stop chasing things that don't align. You stop saying yes to things that drain you. You walk the path that *feels right* for you.

Recap:

Purpose: *A future-facing vision that drives you forward.*
Meaning: *The depth and significance you find in your present and past.*
There will never be a perfect time to pause and find your purpose and meaning. There will always be another carrot dangling in front of you—a job, a promotion, a reason to stay busy on the default path. But you will never find them in convenience. You will only find them by mustering the courage to travel the Unscripted path, *On Purpose!*

Now it's time to pause. Let yourself ask the questions in the framework ahead. Write until the answers make you breathe differently. That will be the beginning of your freedom. And if it feels uncomfortable, then you're doing it right. Discomfort is the doorway, and simply attempting this exercise is already an act of bravery.

The Unscripted Compass:
Discover Your Purpose and Meaning

Finding Your Purpose

→ *Why are you here?*
(Write down your why, then ask why five times to get to its depth.)

→ *What do you hope to have achieved in your life?*
What things would you regret not having done on your deathbed?

You'll know it's your real purpose because it will feel like: *This is it.* Like something you'd long since lost has finally come home. It might take days or weeks to find the answer. But if finding your why gives you the freedom to fulfill your Call to More, isn't that worth the discomfort?

At first, my answers to this exercise were shallow, all about me. But I knew I'd found my purpose the moment I wrote a purpose that went beyond myself: *"To help others find their identity beyond societal expectations and fulfill the dream that the Creator has for them."* That's when I understood why writing this book sometimes brought me to tears of joy: it felt like I was finally living my purpose by contributing to something beyond myself.

Find Your Meaning → *What gives your life depth right now?*

- *What past experiences have shaped you?*
- *What present moments feel rich with connection, beauty, or contribution?*
- *What future memories do you want to create?*
- *How can you create experiences that align with your purpose?*

CHAPTER 17

On Creativity
What Longs to Be Expressed Through You?

Fulfilling your purpose and finding meaning in life will demand that you resurrect that part of you—the creative, expressive self that still remembers how to play and build.

—Katrina Azer

Each of us has a unique talent, and the reason we never feel enough is because we keep looking sideways at everyone else's talent, at everyone else's timeline, instead of leaning into what life is offering us through the lens of our own gifts and our own opportunities. We are so busy scrolling ourselves into numbness that we forget to look at what's right in front of us and the inner potential we've buried under distraction.

When you reconnect with your true identity beyond the script, you'll find what's been buried under the rubble of performative work. Fulfilling your purpose and finding meaning in life will demand that you resurrect that part of you—the creative, expressive self that still remembers how to play and build.

You know that unmistakable lift when you've created something meaningful, whether it's a meal so comforting it silences the table, a canvas that finally captures what your words couldn't say, or a photo that freezes a feeling you didn't want to lose. It is found in that moment when creation meets presence. Don't mistake it for a fluke because creativity is in your DNA.

We were born creatives and artists before we were employees. Our ancestors didn't only hunt and survive; they painted, carved, sang, told stories, and danced. The Lascaux cave paintings in France (over 17,000 years old) prove that creativity was how we made meaning, passed on knowledge, processed emotion, and connected.

We were artists before we were employees.

Look at a child, and you'll see how naturally they are drawn to creativity. They draw, play pretend, build, and imagine. It's only once formal education systems and social norms are imposed that we learn to prioritize utility over expression. In fact, some of the greatest minds in education and innovation have called this out. Sir Ken Robinson's famous TED Talk, *Do Schools Kill Creativity?* makes it painfully clear where the real danger lies in education. As he puts it, "We are educating people out of their creative capacities… I believe this passionately, that we don't grow into creativity; we grow out of it. Or rather, we get educated out of it."[1] If more people tapped back into their inner creative—the part of them that remembers how to build, paint, write, question, and explore—fewer people would feel tethered to "just" having a job.

The concept of fixed jobs didn't solidify until the Industrial Revolution. Before that, people lived in roles that were craft-based, family-taught, or creatively improvisational. The rise of standardized labor created a model where humans became cogs, not creators.

Additionally, a 2022 randomized controlled trial published in the *American Journal of Medicine* showed that creative arts therapies, including visual art, music, writing, and movement, were effective for stress reduction, burnout, emotional regulation, and improved psychological resilience among health professionals.[2]

Creativity is your way to channel emotion, build resilience, and express your experience of life. It is how you express your deepest longings and yearnings, how you reflect on life beyond the material, and how you cope with life's highs and lows. Many writers and artists have echoed that when creativity is not expressed, it feels as if something inside them begins to explode, die, or go numb, as if a part of them shuts down at the expense of expressing their gift.

Finding your gift and your talent will elevate your self-expression. You will become a far better version of yourself—a more life-embracing version of you. Many pharmacists fear discovering their talent, in case they like it more than their job. And to that, I say: There's no reason why your creative endeavor can't become a source of income and complement your "job." I'm still a pharmacist, but I'm also a writer, dancer, blogger, and podcaster. You are a human with talents who happens to "work" as a pharmacist to earn a living. You can contribute to society in more than one way.

If the guilt remains, it means the script is still running. It means you haven't fully detached from the "I am only a pharmacist" identity yet. You must shed that identity and understand that there is more to you. You are an individual with talents and potential that stretch far beyond the white coat. This step is crucial to your Unscripting journey. Every individual has a creative side they must tap into to reach their full potential. I became a far more successful version of myself the moment I tapped into my creativity.

"But I don't know what my talent is," many people say, and it's a fair question. You have to allow yourself to experiment and accept being mediocre at a whole assortment of things before you figure out where your hidden talent might be. You need a few honest attempts before you can decide, and even if you're not naturally good at something, you'll know whether it's enjoyable or something you're willing to keep showing up for.

The system didn't kill your creativity; it buried your creativity under compliance, and now it's time to reclaim it. If time is crushing you, check your phone usage. There's margin hiding there. And there is no better time to find the creative you. This is your permission to pick up that paintbrush, write that article, or cook that recipe that's been sitting on the kitchen bench for months. Don't let this be another action you shake off as unimportant because the act itself is the doorway to creative freedom. Creativity doesn't ask for perfection; it asks only for your presence.

CHAPTER 18

On Spirituality
What Is Calling You Deeper Than Success?

Spirituality is what helps you hold on when the title doesn't.

—Katrina Azer

If identity is the mirror, purpose is the destination, meaning is the journey's depth, and creativity is the expression, then spirituality is the foundation that makes it all sustainable. Therefore, I can't go on without dedicating a specific chapter to spirituality in a book about finding your purpose.

For honesty's sake, I want to declare openly that my own calling centers around my faith in Jesus Christ. I don't expect you to share my faith to find this chapter useful, but I do want you to know the spiritual well I drink from that replenishes my soul and is the reason for my being and purpose, so that you can decide how you wish to drink. If you're curious about how my Christian faith has shaped my journey more explicitly, I've included an appendix at the end of the book for you to explore.

Spirituality is the part of you that seeks connection beyond the surface and beyond the self. It's the quiet knowing that something deeper is guiding you, anchoring you, calling you. It's not about religion, rituals, or rigid belief systems (though for many, it includes them). It's about alignment—a sense that your life is not random. That your purpose is not a goal but a calling. That your gifts are not talents but assignments. Spirituality is what helps you hold on when the title doesn't, when the paycheck doesn't fulfill you, and when the system lets you down. It reminds you: *You were created on purpose, for a purpose.*

Every pharmacist needs a grounding practice, spiritual or otherwise, regardless of whom or what you worship. You need a transcendent experience to connect you to the divine beyond what you can see. You need to be tethered to something beyond you because when all your world falls apart, that's the only thing you've got to keep you sane. Whether you call it God, Source, or Spirit, whether you meditate or simply contemplate the mystery of being alive, what matters is making space to connect with it. Without spirituality, I wouldn't have endured any of the hardships I faced in my career. Spirituality instilled in me the faith needed to keep going in the darkest moments. It gave me hope and endurance.

Spirituality also creates abundance in your life. Connecting with the Source of your being helps you see that there is more to life than the material because the Divine is the source of all that is—the Source of Abundance. And when you seek that type of abundance first—the abundance of the mind and spirit, not money—you get rewarded with all the goodness life offers without even asking for it. That is what I call soul-led alignment. Your soul becomes so attuned and receptive to the abundance of the Divine that your purpose and vision for your life seek beyond the conventional, beyond money-oriented success. You seek meaning in everything you do. You become more intentional in your life and career. You seek beyond the *more* that society convinces you will bring you happiness.

Spirituality also elevates your creative potential. The calm and mindful state brought on by spiritual practices (whether through prayer, meditation, stillness, or reflection) creates space within you. Space to hear, to receive, to imagine. It's in that quiet clarity that you often find yourself reconnected with your most creative, unfiltered self.

And it's in that stillness—when the noise dims and the world's expectations fall quiet—that you hear what's been buried under the performance: your true gifts. Not just your talents and strengths, but God-given grace entrusted to us to serve others with.

There's a verse that once shifted something deep in me and helped me see the connection between spirituality and creativity: "Each of you should use whatever gift you have received to serve others, as faithful stewards of God's grace in its various forms" (1 Peter 4:10).

Suddenly, the things I thought were "just hobbies" or side skills outside pharmacy, such as writing, feel less like hobbies and more like assignments. Spirituality creates the stillness, clarity, and alignment that help you move your gifts from acts of self-expression to *sacred stewardship.* You see your talents not as self-fulfilling activities but as acts of service. And when you use your gifts in service—rooted in love, not striving—what you're actually doing is stewarding grace.

And if you think you are not worthy of exercising that talent—because I know that voice too well, the doubt that whispers, *Who are you to write, to create, to lead?*—know that God doesn't call the qualified. He qualifies the called. You don't have to be good enough or qualified enough for Him. If He only called the qualified, then most of us wouldn't get a look in. Not the pharmacist who failed that one paper and still carries it like shame in their pocket, nor the one who never did a residency but has more wisdom from their twelve-hour shifts than a textbook could ever hold, nor the one who fumbles when speaking but has a voice that could move a room if only they believed it was worth hearing—and certainly not me. It was spirituality that allowed me to walk into rooms I had no business entering, except that God's calling whispered, *Go*, and I obeyed.

Your qualifications don't validate your calling because your calling came first. So if the impostor is louder than your conviction, find that talent and step into it anyway. Trust that what you lack in credentials you'll find in courage, clarity, and divine alignment found in spiritual practice.

This is your permission to pause in stillness, however you practice, and connect with the Divine. Whisper a prayer, sit in silence, watch the wind move through the trees, or simply listen for that deep call. Whatever your tradition, I want to remind you that spirituality isn't about only about religion; it's about making space for the deeper call that refuses to be silenced. Allow yourself to be led by something deeper—by faith, curiosity, and hope.

CHAPTER 19

On Intuition
How Do You Know Which Voice to Trust?

Intuition isn't the ignition; it's the glow that's been burning under the ashes your entire life, waiting for you to listen.

—Katrina Azer

Now that you've remembered who you truly are and identified your purpose, your creativity, and your spirituality, it is time to connect with and reclaim your internal guiding force—your inner voice or intuition.

Many of us don't trust our inner voice enough. For many, the inner critic is louder than our inner voice. Your intuition might feel abstract or ungrounded, and maybe you've never connected with it before. That's why this chapter is the last in the series, because the groundwork had to be done first. When you find your identity, tap into your purpose, and nurture a spiritual connection with the source of abundance, only then can your intuition get loud enough to be heard.

To hear your intuition, you must first understand yourself, be willing to sit in the discomfort of stillness, cultivate internal positive narratives, and practice silencing the inner critic. Intuition is a muscle that grows the more you are attuned to yourself, your thoughts, and your instincts. The more you practice listening to your intuition, the more it becomes a trusted voice and a faithful guide. Every time you follow it, and it leads you somewhere right, you create proof for the next time it speaks. It is a constant journey of self-discovery, of becoming. If you keep shutting it down, if you keep telling yourself, "This is a terrible idea," or "Who do you think you are to do this?" then it gets quieter and quieter until it disappears altogether. You have to talk to it, train it, and respect it.

What I've learned over time is that intuition is *not* meant to make sense. In fact, most of the time it's so illogical that people around you will doubt you because intuition isn't math, where 1 + 1 = 2. It's physics. It's energy. It's the alignment of what you've put out into the world—energy that says, *I am open and allowing all the possibilities that God* (or the universe, Allah, or whatever spiritual force you believe in) *has for me to find me.*

As an example, it didn't make sense for a newbie writer like me to feature in an opinion column usually claimed by people with far more experience, but it happened. I risked rejection, but if I hadn't listened to that inner nudge and sent that first-ever, subpar article, I probably wouldn't have built the confidence to write this book.

Here's the thing: your destiny is not preset. You create your destiny by listening to your intuition. I don't believe it when people say, "It's not meant to be." I believe that *you can mean it to be* if you listen to your intuition. It's like waiting to catch a train. You catch one train early, you arrive at your destination early, and you run into a connection who offers you the job of your dreams. You catch the next train, and you miss the opportunity—same platform, different outcome.

So when the Unscripted path feels too Unscripted—and it will—learn to get quiet and listen to the inner voice. Your intuition only speaks in solitude, far from the noise and hustle of the world and the people around you, who will almost always oppose your intuition because it seems illogical. But you must remember this: intuition is not logic, and it's not supposed to be.

What happens when people you trust, such as close friends and family, oppose your intuition? Here's what I've learned: no one has walked in your shoes or has your lived experience. Your experiences and perspectives have shaped your thinking and decisions, but none of these people have your life experiences; they're speaking from their perspective and their lens, so how could it be that they're more informed about your path when they have not lived your life? They love you deeply, but they can only see through their lens, not yours. Only you know what fits your soul.

And yes—I get it; it is *so hard* to ignore their voices because to them, your choices might look reckless. But that's where you must remember that your intuition is not supposed to make sense to anyone else.

In your career, you will be bombarded with career advice from every direction. Everyone will give you a plan and a framework. Everyone will have a version of "success" they think you should follow. But their advice is based on following a script handed to them, but this is the Unscripted path, remember? The path of no path, so to speak. So if someone tells you to follow their steps, you will not get there by doing what they have done because you are not them. And if you get there, you won't feel fulfilled because the life they've built won't fit your soul and your purpose. The only way you're going to reach your destiny—the only way you're going to find your Call to More—is by listening to your intuition. Listening to your intuition will lead you to the right opportunities, the right people, and the right places that allow you to have experiences that lead to the freedom we spoke of. You don't need to follow anyone else's steps. Your inner voice is your guiding force; it already knows the way. Trust it.

You don't need to follow anyone else's steps.
Your inner voice is your guiding force;
it already knows the way. Trust it.

Intuition isn't the ignition; it's the glow that's been burning under the ashes your entire life, waiting for you to listen. *Intuition is the heartbeat of the Unscripted path.* So now that your intuition calls on you to become *Unscripted On Purpose*, will you listen to its call?

EPILOGUE SERIES

The Unscripted Epilogue Letters

Before I close, there are a few things I didn't say earlier. Not because they didn't matter, but because they revealed themselves only once the story had settled. These truths aren't chapters; they're lessons and reminders that stayed with me long after the shift in the path began.

What follows isn't a linear roadmap. These aren't chapters but letters, reminders, and anchors from my journey. Think of them as field notes from someone who is still walking the Unscripted path, imperfectly but intentionally.

You can return to them when you feel unsure. Let them serve as your anchor when the old script whispers that it would have been easier to stay safe.

LETTER ONE

The Final Unscripting
Letting Go of Who You Are Not

Dear Pharmacist Who Is Ready to Get Unscripted On Purpose,

I know how hard it is to choose the Unscripted path. This might be the awakening you've needed for years, but awakenings don't arrive gently. It's disorienting to peel away an identity you've lived inside for years, especially when you've known no better than the script handed to you—the one tied to the industry's version of success, trying to hit those KPIs or waiting for that next performance review to prove you are enough.

But what if disorientation isn't proof you're lost, but proof you're finally on your way?

Letting go of who you are not is grief work. It is not about abandoning all you were. It is about remembering all that you are before you were a pharmacist. It is remembering that you are called on purpose, for a purpose. Embracing this new direction is a rebirth, so give yourself grace, stay open, and be anchored in the identity that you are beginning to embrace. It is okay to feel lost, confused, cracked open, and overwhelmed while simultaneously inspired and empowered for what's to come. That disorientation is part of your awakening, and you are not required to have it all figured out. It is Unscripted, remember?

The Unscripted Journey isn't a destination. It's a journey of *becoming*. It's something you continue choosing again and again, even on the days you miss the old certainty. Once you glimpse what it feels like to live Unscripted, you can't go back to shrinking.

And though it may feel overwhelming at first—because stability feels safer than expansion—I invite you to wonder what might be possible if you gave yourself permission to be seen for the first time. To travel through life outside the script *On Purpose.* To step into rooms you're told you don't belong in. To own the liberty of choosing what you step into, what you say yes and no to. And to wake to a new day without dread but with the feeling of living a better version of yourself.

If regret lingers over paths not taken, opportunities you missed, or choices you now second-guess, know that you were doing the best you could with what you had at the time. And to that version of you who stayed too long, who didn't speak up, who gave too much, who was trying to survive—thank them for the endurance, because they got you here. And here is enough. The rejections and wrong turns weren't detours; they were directions that brought you here. They brought you back to this page and to yourself.

And if you're still sitting with a silent ache or carrying burdens from the past, maybe this is your sign to put them down. To stop replaying the betrayal, the burnout, or the breakdown. To stop asking for closure and start asking for courage. Don't rush, and don't silence the aches with another productivity hack. Let it breathe, and sit with it long enough to ask: "What is this ache trying to teach me? What version of myself have I been suppressing just to survive?" You do not need to have all the answers yet, but don't abandon the questions.

There is a future you are called to walk into. And you cannot walk freely into it while dragging every regret behind you. The best way to move forward is not by force but by release. To step into the *more,* you must unclench the grip on what was. The past has served its purpose, and now it's time to release it—not because it didn't matter, but because it no longer serves or defines you.

This is not the part where you sprint, but where you exhale. And maybe for the first time in your career, you do not need to perform, achieve, prove, or fix. Maybe all that's asked of you now is simply to pause and listen to your breath, your body, your story, your faith, and begin walking again—not with answers, but with courage. Because your becoming is found in stillness and alignment. And though the path forward is not paved, not perfect, and has no clear map, it is yours.

It has always been embedded within you, waiting for you to stop asking, start trusting, and begin walking in it.
You need to trust yourself as the map.

The journey on that path begins now, by letting go of who you no longer are and embracing the new you.

With love and purpose,

Katrina

LETTER TWO

On Fear
Embracing Discomfort, Rejection, and Risk

Dear Pharmacist Who Is Held from the Unscripted Path by Fear,

To walk the Unscripted path, you will meet the edge of your comfort, the sting of rejection, and the flutter of risk. These are the unspoken tolls at the gate, but if you've done the groundwork—if you've anchored yourself in your identity, your purpose, and your values—these tolls no longer feel like threats; they feel like invitations.

Most pharmacists don't talk about fear. We disguise it as professionalism, bury it under logic, and say, "I'm not ready," when what we mean is, "I am scared." But behind every discomfort, rejection, and risk lives fear. And the only way to Unscript yourself is to walk toward it.

To follow your purpose beyond the script, you will need to do things that don't guarantee a safe outcome. You will need to say yes when you want to scream no. You will need to risk your reputation, your comfort, and your certainty. That guitar class means leaving work early and enduring your manager's side-eye. That job application you keep avoiding. That article you never posted. These aren't career moves; they are character builders.

And just like intuition, they are muscles that strengthen with use. The more you stretch them, the more they will serve you. Everything you want—every meaningful outcome you crave—sits on the other side of fear.

I've been stretched by discomfort, undone by rejection, and carved open by risk so many times that I no longer run from them. I allow them and write through them. This book is the overcoming of fear in action.

On Discomfort...

Discomfort is a directional sign, a signal that you are growing. Comfort is sameness. It is doing the same thing each day, seeing the same outcomes, and holding onto the same patterns. It is predictable, but it is also numbing. Discomfort signals growth because you're doing something that pushes your boundaries.

Think of it this way: the burn of your first few workouts, the ache in your arms when you lift again after months off, or the discomfort of studying for that pharmacy degree, those sleepless nights, those first shaky dispensary shifts. You endured that discomfort because you knew what it would yield. The discomfort of trying something new—of letting yourself be clumsy at it for a while, of not being instantly good—is exactly what you need because this is your becoming phase.

When you step onto your Unscripted path, expect discomfort. In fact, welcome it. You'll find it in small things, like staying in the conversation when you usually slip away or putting your hand up when the old version of you would've stayed quiet. These are micro-movements of Unscripting. They are not loud, but they are transformational. You don't desensitize discomfort by avoiding it. You desensitize it by meeting it.

On Rejection...

You will be declined. You will be walked out on. You will face rejection in all its forms, some sharp and sudden, others quiet and slow-burning—the kind that lingers longer than you'd care to admit. Threads of rejection stitch together the book you're holding. Rejection from people I trusted. From the systems I tried to change. From projects I poured my soul into, only to watch them unravel.

All of those experiences hurt deeply. But in that ache, you hear something louder, a whisper that says, *Do it anyway.* Sometimes it takes the finality of a rejection for you to take tangible action. Sometimes the door that slams shut is the only way you'll notice the window that's been open all along.

You will face rejection in work, in love, and in life. And while it will always sting, it is not a statement of your worth. It's often a rerouting—a sacred detour, and a disguised redirection toward the thing that's actually meant for you. You might not see what's waiting behind the next door yet, but I promise that if you keep walking and keep trusting God and your intuition, you'll find that the door that finally opens is the one that was always meant to be yours.

On Risk...

We take risks every day, but we don't always name them as such. Walking out your front door and assuming you'll return safely? That is a risk. Speaking up in a meeting where your voice has long been dismissed? Risk. Saying no to the stable job that's been draining the life out of you, even when you don't have a backup yet? That is a risk too. But here's the difference between ordinary and extraordinary lives: those who live Unscripted not only tolerate risk; they trust it.

And trust doesn't mean recklessness. It means discernment. It means taking calculated risks and knowing that if the outcome doesn't land exactly where you'd hoped, you still have the resilience and creativity to pivot.

Risk is meaningless without conviction and belief. It's easy to flirt with change when the stakes are low, but it's conviction that carries you when the outcome is unclear. And faith in your ability to learn, rebuild, and create something from scratch if you have to. Risk—held by conviction and belief—is what aligns you.

It may not be the formula for overnight success, but it is one for a soul-led, aligned movement. Getting Unscripted means leaning into the awkwardness, into the uncertainty, into the terrifying thrill of not knowing what comes next and choosing to walk anyway, remembering that the Unscripted path was never meant to be safe. *It was only ever the true path.*

Yours in embracing fear,

Katrina

LETTER THREE

On Curiosity
Let It Be Your Compass

Dear Pharmacist Who Doesn't Ask Enough Questions,

What if you stopped asking, "Can I do this?" and started asking, "What happens if I try?" Curiosity is the first crack on the path to getting *Unscripted On Purpose.* It's the soft but seismic question that asks, "What if there's more?" Once you ask this question, the status quo loosens its grip on you.

I never sat with *what-ifs* in my career; I answered them. Every meaningful shift I've made—every pivot, reinvention, and breakthrough—began with a single question I wasn't afraid to follow. Early on, I traded the illusion of control for the wonder of exploration. I became someone who asked too many questions, enough to unnerve those still clinging to the script. And when the answer came back as, "*This is how we've always done it,*" I took that as a dare.

Curiosity was a spark. It was tiny, inconvenient and dangerous to those guarding the old script, who were annoyed by my questions. But once lit, it changed my direction, and I couldn't unsee the truth it revealed. I allowed that spark to become my compass, drawing me toward the unexplored, toward everything I was forbidden to want, toward the identity beyond the title, and toward what hadn't been tried yet.

Curiosity precedes fear. First, the question arises, then fear tries to silence it, and that's when the test begins. If you silence the fear, listen to your intuition, brave the question, and follow it, you strengthen your intuition. But if you dismiss it, mute the wondering, and accept a "this is just how things are" mindset, you dull it. Over time, you forget how to ask, how to wonder, and how to hear yourself.

To be curious is to believe in possibility and to embrace imagination. Everything around you began with a question. A thought in someone's head turned into a hypothesis, which turned into action. When you believe in possibility, you don't feel confined to the norm. You know there is something more. Even if you don't know *what* it is yet, you trust that it's waiting to be found by the one who dares to ask. It opens doors that credentials or qualifications cannot. When I began my writing journey, I didn't stop when I told myself, *But I don't have a literature degree.* Instead, I changed my thoughts: *I wonder what the editor will think of my article.* I didn't attach myself to the outcome; I wasn't writing to impress but to get feedback and learn.

One of our biggest weaknesses as pharmacists is our perfectionist tendencies, but curiosity is your antidote. This is your one-way ticket out of the perfectionism loop. Allow yourself to ask more questions. To explore the *what-ifs.* To stop taking anything (especially systems, job descriptions, or old ways of working) at face value. Staying trapped in perfectionism is the enemy of the good, which is better than perfect. Perfection often leads to paralysis for fear of failure, but curiosity leads to movement. And when you allow yourself to try, even if you fail, you will fail forward and come out a few steps ahead of where you once stood, but never back where you began.

So dare to explore, to try and fail, to ask the questions. Because to ask is to be curious, and to be curious is to believe in possibility and in your intuition—the internal guiding force that will always lead you to the awakened, alive version of yourself, living *Unscripted On Purpose.*

With love and purpose,

Katrina

LETTER FOUR

On Leadership
Leading from Identity, Not Ambition

Dear Pharmacist Who Seeks to Be a Leader,

In the last letter, I called you to be led by curiosity. Curiosity, when followed long enough, will eventually lead you to a crossroad of insight and responsibility. Because once you start seeing what's broken, you can't unsee it. And once you start asking the bold questions, you may find yourself being called to answer them—out loud, in front of others, with more courage than you think you have.

One of the most impactful ways to Unscript is to lead, to become a trusted, grounded voice, because you are now moved by purpose, by a calling that pulls you toward service beyond yourself. True leadership is legacy, and legacy is never built on self-preservation; it is built on service to others.

Most pharmacists confuse leadership with plain advocacy. Their logic says: *If I apply to be appointed to this advocacy board, I'll be seen as a leader. I'll speak on behalf of pharmacists. I'll uplift the profile of the profession. And I'll finally have influence.* But this is performative leadership. It is title-seeking, role-chasing, and leading from optics rather than alignment.

Authentic leadership isn't something you're appointed to; it's something you embody. It doesn't wait for the committee to approve the agenda. It doesn't need a platform to act with conviction. Leadership is lived long before it is recognized.

Leadership is not a badge you wear or a role you apply for. It doesn't seek to be seen or praised. Instead, it responds to a need; it serves without waiting for permission; it allows you to do the work that aligns with who you are and who you're called to become.

Leadership is the decision to take responsibility in the very moments others look away, when silence is safer, when apathy is easier, and when waiting for someone else to act feels more comfortable than stepping forward into the unknown. It's deciding to be the change you so desperately wish existed. To advocate when no one is looking, behind closed doors and publicly. In quiet meetings and uncomfortable conversations. In forums where it's easy to stay silent, and in moments when your voice might cost you. Speaking your truth will sometimes earn you criticism, silence, or subtle punishment. And yes, some will dislike you, misunderstand you, and even target you. But still, you speak, because the long-term impact of aligned, respectful truth-telling always outweighs the short-term discomfort of disapproval.

Leaders are the people who show up in the darkest days. They show up with intention, care, and attention that says, "This matters." They choose to do the right thing, especially when the wrong thing is easier, faster, and often rewarded. From early in my career, I listened to the quiet nudge of leadership. Not because I was trying to rebel or disrupt authority, but because I couldn't silence that inner voice that whispered when something wasn't right. It was easy to dismiss that forged prescription. The easier path would have been to obey, to keep my head down, to earn the nod of approval, but I listened to my intuition and asked the hard question. Obedience would've earned me comfort, but integrity earned me a recommendation letter that opened the door to leadership.

So, dear pharmacist, if you feel called to lead, don't chase titles or wait for appointments. Don't confuse leadership with hierarchy. Leadership has never been about positions; it's about leading from service, speaking from purpose, and acting with intention.

When you lead from intention and not ambition, you leave trust, healing, and courage in the hearts of those you've served. You will feel lighter, steadier, no longer hustling for approval but anchored in the quiet knowing that your leadership mattered.

No one needs permission to become a leader. What you need is belief in the voice that already lives inside you: the voice of integrity, alignment, and intention. This is what it means to lead with legacy. To influence with grace. And to live out leadership, *On Purpose.*

With love and purpose,

Katrina

LETTER FIVE

On Consistency
The Sacred Practice of Showing Up

Dear Pharmacist Who Struggles to Show Up,

It's time to come full circle with *Unscripting On Purpose* because no Unscripted life is ever fully lived without the sacred, repeated act of showing up—for yourself and for others.

You cannot step into the Call to More if you don't show up for it. Showing up is the quiet engine of consistency. It is doing what must be done even when everything inside you is screaming *don't*. To show up in discomfort. To show up despite rejection. To show up even when leadership feels lonely. Showing up says: *I will stay true to the Unscripting, no matter how I'm feeling.*

Showing up when all you want to do is hide from the world. When there is disapproval at work, when there's a target on your back, when your motives are misunderstood and your voice misread, and still you show up anyway because living Unscripted requires giving up the approval of others.

Perhaps the most challenging thing about showing up is feeling unappreciated and unseen when you do, and yet you keep showing up anyway. You don't do it because you're chasing appreciation (though that's always validating), but because it aligns with your values—because not showing up would leave you feeling off, guilty, or disconnected from yourself. You show up because it is who you are; it is an act of devotion, not just duty.

To show up fully, with intention and purpose for others, you must first show up for yourself. You don't need permission to show up for yourself—to take that yoga class, to cancel that meeting, to choose rest instead. You don't need to justify why rest matters or explain to anyone why solitude feels holy. I used to believe that self-care was selfish. I wore exhaustion and productivity like a badge of honor. But after I burned out, I changed everything. I became selfish (radically so) about my well-being. That way, my cup is always full and abundant, and I can give more. Showing up isn't just about being dependable for others; it's about not ghosting yourself. Because there is a cost to not showing up for yourself; it manifests as distraction, overwork, or avoidance of everything and everyone, even those closest to you.

Without showing up, especially in the hard seasons, the hollow mornings, the days when everything in you wants to crawl back under the covers and opt out, you can't become the Unscripted version of you. Showing up *is* the becoming, and you can't disappear from the process that's shaping you. It is the driving force that moves you forward when the road ahead feels blurry or unbearable. It is the engine of the Unscripted path, and without it, the path fades, and you risk defaulting back to the script you swore you'd never return to—the one that asked you to shrink, to conform, to abandon who you truly are.

Consistency in showing up does not have to be perfect. That's the lie we're sold—the filtered illusion that everyone else is doing it flawlessly, that they never miss a step, never skip a beat, never fall apart behind the scenes. But it's okay to miss a day (or ten!). That's not failure; that's being human. Because consistency isn't rigid discipline; it means returning to alignment after drifting. It's reconnecting with your soul after the chaos and pausing long enough to hear your intuition again.

So, if the world tells you that you've failed to show up, allow your own evidence to silence that voice. The evidence of the days you showed up when it was raining inside your chest. When you showed up with grief in your mouth and a head heavier than a rock.

Some days, showing up looks like submitting the grant application. On other days, it looks like canceling the meeting or saying no to your boss. And sometimes it means saying yes to your child when they ask you to go outside and watch the sky. Sacred consistency isn't grand. It's grounded. And grounding allows you to grow.

So many times, I wanted to walk away from this book. And not just wanted to—I *did.* Days when my fingers rested on the keyboard, every part of me heavy with inertia. And yet, it was those quiet DMs—the ones from pharmacists I'd never met—that pulled me back. The ones that said, "I'm waiting for your words." That was when I showed up, even on the days when showing up felt like a fight. I pushed myself to write. Just one word. Then the next. Line after line. Chapter after chapter. I kept going until I got there.

Showing up is hard. Excruciating on some days. But the reward—that whisper that says, *This is good. This feels true despite how hard it is*—is worth it.

This is what it means to live *Unscripted On Purpose.* It is not about living perfectly, but persistently. Not for applause, but with intention and alignment with the Call to More. And when the road feels blurry, when no one is clapping, and when the next step feels impossible, show up anyway because the you that you are becoming is waiting on the other side of that moment. It is in showing up that the becoming happens, that you continue to live *Unscripted On Purpose.*

Yours faithfully and *On Purpose,*

Katrina

Final Echo

I didn't write this book as someone who has it all figured out but as someone still walking the Unscripted journey in real time, discovering that there is a whole series of truths to unearth, questions to wrestle with, experiences to live, and an identity to uncover beneath it all. I wrote it because choosing to take this journey gave me the freedom I've been longing for, and I hope it's the same for you, too. This purpose-driven book is in service of you—the pharmacist who is becoming, who has already begun the journey of getting *Unscripted On Purpose.*

I pray that through unearthing your identity, mapping your purpose and meaning, listening to your intuition, choosing curiosity over silence, and transcending with spirituality, you find your Call to More. It isn't a roar. It doesn't announce itself with certainty, clarity, or control. It arrives slowly. In the ache that builds after too many silent commutes. In the pull that won't leave, even when the next role looks good on paper. It starts in the exhaustion you can't explain. In the whisper that says, *Maybe I'm meant for something else,* which gets louder every time you try to pretend you can't hear it.

It doesn't come with a job title. It doesn't wait for your next credential, and it won't be delivered in an email or a neatly worded offer. The Call to More comes when you decide that your purpose, your voice, your story, your talent, and your truth can no longer be delayed. This is the liberation you've been waiting for—the permission to move forward on the path that honors both your soul and your science.

This is your new beginning—*Unscripted On Purpose.*

My Dear Pharmacist,

You are Called to More beyond the script.

A dream is waiting for you. Just waiting for you to step into it. One so soaked in purpose and alignment, it won't only fulfill your career; it will also nourish your soul. So don't tiptoe toward it. Run toward the more with faith, not fear. Run with trust that the One who called you will not leave you unfinished.

This is the moment you stop waiting for permission or the map. Your inner voice knows the way, so trust it.

Right here, right now, is the reinvention of the truest version of you. The version found in the path that doesn't promise ease or clarity but will always feel like truth. And when the world hands you its script again, tear it up and choose the path that was always yours because you are not finished, not silenced, and not small.

You are becoming.

Now, embrace your Call to More.

And live fully. Unscripted On Purpose.

ACKNOWLEDGMENTS

Gratitude for the Hands, Doors, and Detours That Held This Book

To the doors that closed, you made space for better ones to open.

To the endings that barreled in like freight trains,
you lifted me to higher platforms.

To the relationships that broke down,
you made space for better ones to flourish.

To the breakdowns and rock-bottom moments,
you reshaped and reinvented me.

To the rejections that broke me, you reset my compass north.
I'm grateful for the clarity.

And to the old version of me:
Thank you for your courage, endurance,
and for choosing to be Unscripted On Purpose.

I extend my deepest gratitude to the hand that held me together when I couldn't get another word on paper, when self-doubt hissed that I should walk away—Jesus Christ, the Creator, the Source of all that is. My only source of truth: thank you for the peace that surpasses understanding and the courage to keep on this path. Thank you for renewed mercies every morning. Without you, I wouldn't be here.

To every pharmacist who ever wondered, *Is this it*—and kept showing up anyway—this gratitude extends to you. Thank you for embracing this journey and for reading this book. You are the reason this book exists and the reason I show up every day.

To Rachel Firebaugh, Justin Cole, Kay Dunkley, Julie Doan, and Ayomide Ogundipe: thank you for sacrificing your time and heart to beta-read this book. I am deeply indebted to your generosity and candor.

To my mom and dad: you are my angels on earth. You stood by me in the toughest times and never once doubted my adventures and risks, and your unwavering belief in every decision I made empowered me to get here. May God bless you with health and abundance always.

To my daughters: despite my imperfect mothering, you have shown patience and grace. Thank you for enduring the disruptions of this writing life. I love you.

To my brother: thank you for being a rock when everything felt like rubble and for trusting your own brave path. There is nothing better than a creative, adventurous ally.

To Todd Eury and the Pharmacy Podcast Network: thank you for believing in my voice, giving it a platform, and carrying it beyond our shores long before this book existed.

To every owner, manager, colleague, and mentor whose conversations, opportunities, and—yes—detours shaped my journey: thank you. Your noes became necessary signposts.

Last but not least, to my publishing team: Jenna Schrader for thoughtful, exacting developmental edits, and Alan Hebel for the beautiful, heart-forward design. This book is better because of you.

APPENDIX - MY FAITH

For Those Curious About My Faith

I wrote this book for those who feel called to more but don't yet have the words to define it. Some have asked where the language I use—the way I articulate the concepts and how they manifest in my life and career—comes from. The short answer is *my Christian faith.* So, if you're curious to learn more, here's the framework I live by; if not, feel free to skip this part.

The Gospel in Four Movements

1. **Creation**

   God created us in His image on purpose and for a purpose. One only needs to look around at the extraordinary way the universe moves in such order to sense that our existence is beyond mere coincidence—that a Divine Force deliberately and perfectly crafted this beauty beyond our comprehension, a Force that loves mankind and desires our company.

   He gave us dignity, freedom, and stewardship over everything but one thing: He forbade us to eat from the tree of knowledge. Unfortunately, our desire for the wrong "more" made us seek beyond what He offered.

2. **The Fall**

   Despite His warning that whoever eats from the tree would die, we ate of it anyway. We listened—and to this day continue to listen—to what feeds the body, not the soul. We consumed the material, thinking it would fill us, make us powerful, and answer our questions and desires. We ate from the tree and felt the fracture, the disconnection from Him. We were cast out of Eden and wandered the Earth seeking more of the material, building empires, acquiring kingdoms, fighting and killing for power, and we still do. But He didn't leave us to dwell in our misery. He loved us despite our betrayal of His Word.

3. **Redemption**
   God sent His only begotten Son, Jesus Christ, becoming flesh like us, to bear the consequence on our behalf. He paid the price by dying for us on the cross and then conquered death after three days, thereby granting us everlasting life with Him. In that, He restored our relationship with Him. He forgave us so that we may forgive others. He gave us grace so that we may provide it to others. He redeemed us despite our iniquities, and through His wounds we are healed each day.

4. **Restoration**
   Through the mending of this broken relationship, God calls us to live a life that upholds faith and the truth that can only be found in Him—not out of dictatorship, but because when we don't live a life of faith, we suffer more than anything. Faith gives us hope beyond the pains of this world; it steadies us when our world falters. He calls us to love one another as He loves us because love is healing. It brings justice and calm to our shattered world until one day He arrives again in the Second Coming to make all things new—a new heaven and a new earth, free from sorrow and despair.

How This Shaped My Journey

It is through faith that we can survive the harsh realities of a world that chases the material and never feels it is enough. Throughout my Unscripted journey, I walked by faith and not by sight. I knew and believed He had a calling for me; sometimes I listened, and sometimes I didn't. When I didn't, the Holy Spirit that Jesus gifted us with awakened me.

God created us as humans before we were given titles. In fact, He loved man so much that He gave us authority over everything in the Garden of Eden to participate in the creation process with Him, naming everything on Earth. His instruction upon our departure from Eden was to "work to live," not the other way around. Our calling goes beyond our profession; it permeates every aspect of our existence and longs for purpose. That's why the more we chase the material, the more we continue to chase, and the emptier we feel. Our Call to More is relational, toward Him. It is through Him that we find the eternal fulfillment and peace that surpasses understanding.

I found it through suffering, through hardships, through burnout, and through grief. God does not punish us; that is never His intention. He allows holy pauses through different means: through broken relationships, a layoff, the moments you're standing with your hands on your head at the dispensing bench, so that we might seek Him, correct course, and find our real purpose in Him. Sometimes that purpose is found by coming back to who we are beyond the title—the creatives, the preachers, the artists, the writers, the speakers—unearthing the seed He planted in us to serve His kingdom, to not only become more alive in Him, but also to bring more people to Him. That's why we flourish when we do what comes naturally to us (our talent) versus only doing what we feel we have to do to sustain a living (our profession). And I hope that through sharing my Unscripted path, I have shown you how the two can coexist in harmony to serve God's calling in your life.

We are called to serve His purpose in our lives, and when we do, we feel more connected to Him, and we experience the fulfillment we seek. We are called to serve the world with the integrity and compassion He instilled in us, to give more than we take, just as He gave Himself up for us. We are called to restoration and renewal in Him every day, because it is through this daily renewal that we experience a true transformation that not only keeps our faith alive, but also gives us the courage to take the path that is *Unscripted On His Purpose* in our life, ultimately giving us the real joy we long for.

A Quiet Prayer

If you're in that space where you're lacking clarity and direction, where you want to find God but don't know if He is true, where you want to believe but still need evidence, here is a short prayer: *God, if You are truly there, if You want me to believe in You, then show Yourself. Let me experience Your presence in my life today. Amen.*

(If you want to learn more about Jesus, I recommend you read the NIV Bible.)

Closing Blessing

I pray that you find the peace that surpasses all understanding, and that you find the courage to travel the path that is *Unscripted On Purpose.*

With gratitude to Justin Cole, PharmD, for suggesting and reviewing this appendix.

NOTES

Chapter 4 - You Are Not Your Mistakes

1. Brené Brown, *The Gifts of Imperfection: Let Go of Who You Think You're Supposed to Be and Embrace Who You Are* (Center City, MN: Hazelden, 2010)

Chapter 6 - Your Worth Is Not Measured by Their Insecurities

1. Oprah Winfrey, *What I Know For Sure* (New York: Flatiron Books, 2014).

Chapter 7 - You Are Called to Purpose-Soaked Excellence

1. Oprah Winfrey, commencement address, University of Southern California Annenberg School for Communication and Journalism, May 11, 2018. Coverage in ABC News, "Oprah Winfrey dishes out life advice in her USC commencement speech," May 11, 2018.
2. Eckhart Tolle, *A New Earth: Awakening to Your Life's Purpose* (New York: Penguin Group, 2005).

Chapter 13 - Your Call to More Is Unscripted On Purpose

1. Bronnie Ware, *The Top Five Regrets of the Dying: A Life Transformed by the Dearly Departing* (Carlsbad, CA: Hay House, 2011).

Chapter 14 - The Call to More

1. Vinh Giang, interview by Steven Bartlett, "The Public Speaking Expert: This Speaking Mistake Makes People Ignore You! These Small Mistakes Make You Unlikeable!", *The Diary of a CEO with Steven Bartlett* podcast, March 10, 2025.
2. Oprah Winfrey, *What I Know For Sure* (New York: Flatiron Books, 2014).

Chapter 16 - On Purpose & Meaning

1. Martin Luther King Jr., "The Drum Major Instinct," sermon, Ebenezer Baptist Church, Atlanta, GA, February 4, 1968, in *A Knock at Midnight: Inspiration from the Great Sermons of Reverend Martin Luther King, Jr.* (New York: Warner Books, 1998).

Chapter 17 - On Creativity

1. Sir Ken Robinson, "Do Schools Kill Creativity?", TED Talk, Monterey, CA, February 2006, transcript available at TED.com.
2. Marc Moss et al., "The Effect of Creative Arts Therapy on Psychological Distress in Health Care Professionals," *The American Journal of Medicine* 135, no. 10 (2022): 1255–1262.e5. doi:10.1016/j.amjmed.2022.04.016.

www.ingramcontent.com/pod-product-compliance
Lightning Source LLC
LaVergne TN
LVHW100305210926
848480LV00003B/1029
* 9 7 8 1 0 6 7 1 1 9 5 9 1 *